Parenteral and Enteral
Nutrition for Nurses

Parenteral and Enteral Nutrition for Nurses

K. MOGHISSI

BSc, MD, FRCS (Ed), Académie de Chirurgie (Paris), FRCS (Eng)

Consultant Cardio-Thoracic Surgeon
Humberside Cardio-Thoracic Surgical Centre, Hull, N. Humberside

JENNIFER R.P. BOORE

SRN, SCM, RNT, BSc.(Hons), Ph.D.

Lecturer in Nursing Studies
University of Hull, N. Humberside

William Heinemann Medical Books Ltd
London

First published by William Heinemann Medical Books Ltd
23 Bedford Square, London, WC1B 3HH, 1983

ISBN 0-433-22130-5

Filmset in 'Monophoto' Plantin by Eta Services (Typesetters) Ltd, Beccles, Suffolk
and printed by Redwood Burn Ltd, Trowbridge, Wiltshire

Contents

Acknowledgements

We wish to express our gratitude to Mrs M. Dench, Mrs E. Edmond and Mrs J. Pearson, research assistants at the Cardio-Thoracic Surgical Centre, Castle Hill Hospital, Cottingham.

The photographs were prepared by Mr G. Whitehead, Medical Illustration Department, Hull Royal Infirmary and Mr M. Whitlock, Castle Hill Hospital, Cottingham. The artwork was drawn by Miss Carolyn Fussey. We are grateful to them.

We received much advice from the nursing staff of Castle Hill Hospital; in particular Miss E. Cook, the Training Sister, to whom we extend our thanks.

Many painstaking hours were given to typing the manuscript by Mrs C. Scott and Miss Anne Gardham, Castle Hill Hospital, Cottingham, this is much appreciated.

Preface

Recent advances in clinical nutrition, and specifically in artificial feeding, have made a significant contribution to the care of seriously ill patients. However, the full potential benefit lies in the more widespread application of these techniques. This depends on an understanding of the indications for such therapy and knowledge of the technical aspects of parenteral and enteral feeding by all those involved in patient management.

Nurses occupy a primary position in this respect by the very nature of their intimate involvement in patient care. Whatever equipment is used or nutritional programme planned, and whatever the organization developed to deal with the nutritional support of patients, nurses are inevitably closely involved. They are concerned not only with the care of the patient and the artificial feeding system, but also with the organization and the ordering of equipment. This second level of involvement explains some of the detail given in this book of equipment and nutrient solutions available at present.

Underlying the application of artificial feeding to the care of patients is an understanding of normal nutrition. Therefore, the first section of this book considers in some detail the nutrients required in the diet, and the way in which they are metabolized within the body in health. Some of the metabolic disturbances which are found in patients requiring artificial nutrition are also discussed. Nutritional assessment of patients and the methods of artificial feeding have been discussed in some detail. Throughout this volume a particular effort has been made to emphasize the nursing management of the patient receiving artificial feeding.

This book has no claim to be entirely original, but accommodates in one volume material obtained from a variety of sources, together with the personal experience of the authors. It is intended primarily as a practical guide to parenteral and enteral feeding for nurses. However, it is hoped that it will also be of value to medical students and young doctors involved in the management of patient care at ward level.

SECTION I

Metabolism and Nutrients

This section acts as an introduction to artificial feeding. It aims to give a clear understanding of body metabolism and the nutrients required for normal functioning. Diet in health is considered, as well as the metabolic changes which occur under conditions of starvation and following trauma, including surgery. This knowledge is essential to appreciate the importance of artificial feeding considered in later sections.

1. Metabolism

The structural integrity and continued functioning of the body depends on the availability of the energy needed for basic maintenance of the biological machinery, for activity and repair. The constancy of the size, weight and composition of the body results from continued breakdown and resynthesis of body components. The energy required for these reactions is derived from food.

Food is defined as 'any solid or fluid which when swallowed can supply any of the following':

- Material from which the body can produce movement, heat, or other forms of energy.
- Material for growth, repair or reproduction.
- Substances necessary to regulate the production of energy or the processes of growth and repair. (Ministry of Agriculture, Fisheries and Food, 1976.)

Some foods are the major sources of energy (fats and carbohydrates), others are body-building for growth and repair (proteins), while others are necessary for regulation of activities and are known as protective foods (the vitamins). However, these divisions are not absolute as there is some overlapping of these functions.

In the alimentary tract, digestion breaks down the large food molecules into simpler substances, nutrients, which are absorbed across the wall of the gastrointestinal tract into the internal compartment of the body.

Within the body some of these simple compounds—glucose (from carbohydrates), fatty acids (from fats) and amino acids (from proteins)—are gradually broken down into carbon dioxide (CO_2), water (H_2O) and nitrogen-containing substances. These changes release energy which is then stored in the high-energy molecule, adenosine triphosphate (ATP), to be made available for various body activities. The processes by which molecules are broken down into smaller substances and energy is released are, together, known as catabolism. Anabolism, on the other hand, consists of the synthesis of complex structural or storage materials from the simpler compounds, and requires the expenditure of energy (Fig. 1.1).

Metabolism is the sum of the chemical reactions taking place within

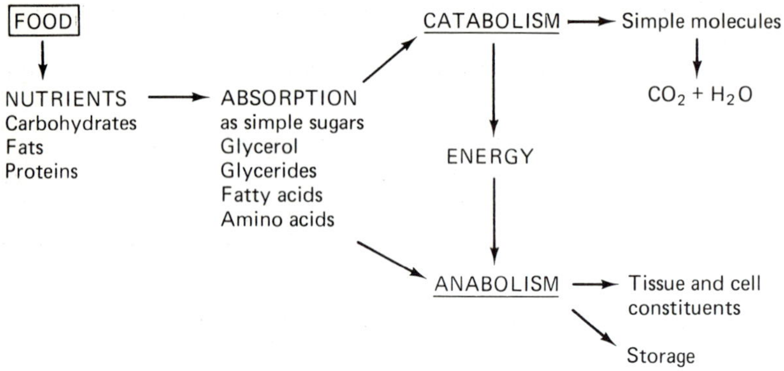

Fig. 1.1 Food, nutrients and metabolism.

the body and includes anabolism and catabolism. The central theme in metabolism is the availability of energy from food, and the utilization of this energy in anabolism.

The energy utilized by the body in maintenance, repair and activity must be supplied by food intake. It is therefore necessary to estimate the energy expenditure of the body. This is done by direct or indirect methods. Normal values of energy required for basal metabolism (i.e. the energy utilized by a person at rest, in a warm room, and at least 12 hours after eating) can be measured, as well as energy expenditure at different levels of activity. This information has been used as a guide to energy requirements for an individual of a particular age and gender by the DHSS (Table 1.3, p. 34). However, people do vary considerably and a more accurate estimation of metabolic rate is required in order to adjust nutrient intake.

The direct method of estimation of metabolic rate was originally carried out by putting an individual in a sealed chamber and measuring the energy value of the food ingested, excreta produced and heat lost from the body. It was found that the energy expended was equivalent to the energy value of food eaten. It also became clear that the energy expenditure was almost directly proportional to the amount of oxygen utilized; 4.83 kcal (20 kJ) of energy is expended for every litre of oxygen used. This is the basis for the indirect measures of metabolic rate, when oxygen utilization is measured at different levels of activity. Studies of metabolic rate show that total energy expenditure for any individual depends on three factors:

1. The energy required for basal metabolism maintains normal body functioning while at rest.

2. The energy needed for physical activity, which is added to the above.

3. The energy used as a result of the specific dynamic action of food. After a meal, the metabolic rate may increase by up to 30%, with protein foods causing the greatest rise, possibly due to the energy involved in digestion, absorption and utilization of the nutrients (Martin, Mayes and Rodwell, 1981).

The central pathway by which energy is made available to the body cells is through the Krebs' cycle (otherwise known as the citric acid cycle or tricarboxylic acid cycle) (Fig. 1.2). Products of fat, glucose and amino acid breakdown can all feed into this cycle and be used for

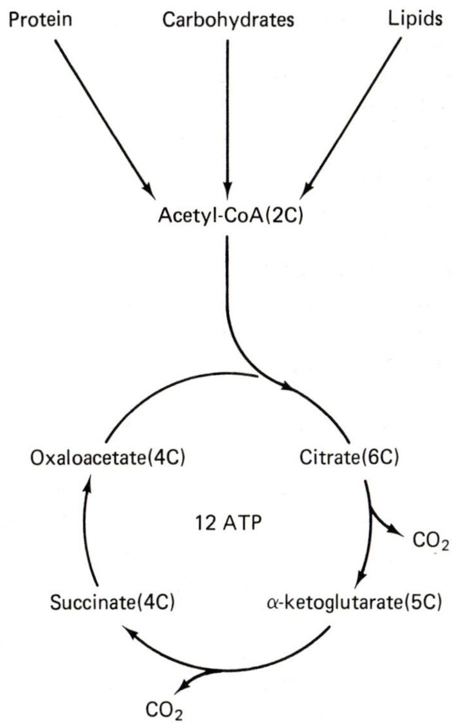

Fig. 1.2 Summary of the Krebs' cycle.

energy production. The major substance feeding into the Krebs' cycle is acetyl coenzyme-A—a 2-carbon molecule combined with coenzyme-A.

Figure 1.2 illustrates the Krebs' cycle in which the 2-carbon molecule combines with a 4-carbon molecule to form a 6-carbon molecule (citrate). This then passes through a series of chemical reactions in which 2 molecules of carbon dioxide (CO_2) are released and 2 water molecules are formed. In a single cycle, 12 molecules of ATP are formed from 1 acetate molecule. The Krebs' cycle can only function in the presence of oxygen.

CARBOHYDRATES

These are composed of carbon, hydrogen and oxygen with the general formula of $C_n(H_2O)_n$.

Man's diet contains a mixture of carbohydrates, the commonest being monosaccharides, disaccharides and polysaccharides.

Monosaccharides

These include hexoses, containing 6 carbon atoms in the molecule, e.g. glucose, fructose, galactose and pentoses, which are 5-carbon molecules.

Disaccharides

These are formed from 2 monosaccharides, and are digested into these before absorption. The three main disaccharides in the diet are maltose (2 molecules of glucose); lactose (1 molecule of glucose, 1 molecule of galactose); and sucrose (1 molecule of glucose, 1 molecule of fructose).

Polysaccharides

These are formed by the condensation of many monosaccharide units. The most important polysaccharide in the diet to supply nutrients is starch, which is found in potatoes, bread, etc. Cellulose is another polysaccharide ingested in large quantities, but which cannot be digested by human beings. However, it provides fibre or roughage in the diet.

Glycogen is the storage form of carbohydrate in animals and found in very small amounts in the diet.

Carbohydrate metabolism

The end products of carbohydrate digestion in the gastrointestinal tract are monosaccharides, of which glucose is the most important.

Monosaccharides are absorbed partly by simple diffusion through the intestinal wall, but glucose is absorbed mainly by active transport. In active transport, energy is used and the substances being absorbed are moved from an area where they are in low concentration, to an area of high concentration. The absorbed monosaccharides are transferred via the venous portal system to the liver, where galactose and fructose are converted to glucose.

Most of the body tissues use a variety of substances for energy, but the brain in particular can (under normal circumstances) only utilize glucose as an energy source. It is therefore essential that the blood glucose is maintained within normal limits* (3.3–5.5 mmol/l) at all times. Thus, the way in which glucose and other substances are metabolized varies in relation to nutrient intake.

After a meal, the blood glucose level rises and then, over a period of about 2 hours, falls in response to the action of insulin. During this period, glucose may be disposed of in a number of ways (Fig. 1.3):

1. Glucose is broken down through the glycolysis pathway (Fig. 1.3) when a series of chemical reactions converts glucose to 2-, 3-carbon molecules and eventually to pyruvate. Pyruvate enters the mitochondria (powerhouses) of the cell and is converted to acetyl-CoA molecules, resulting in the net formation of 14 ATP molecules. This is added to the ATP formed in the Krebs' cycle (Fig. 1.2) by the metabolism of 2 acetyl-CoA molecules. Thus, under aerobic conditions, 38 molecules of ATP are formed from the breakdown of 1 glucose molecule. However, under anaerobic conditions, pyruvate is converted to lactate (which is reconverted to glucose in the liver) with the net formation of only 2 molecules of ATP from 1 molecule of

* The blood glucose results vary slightly according to the method used.

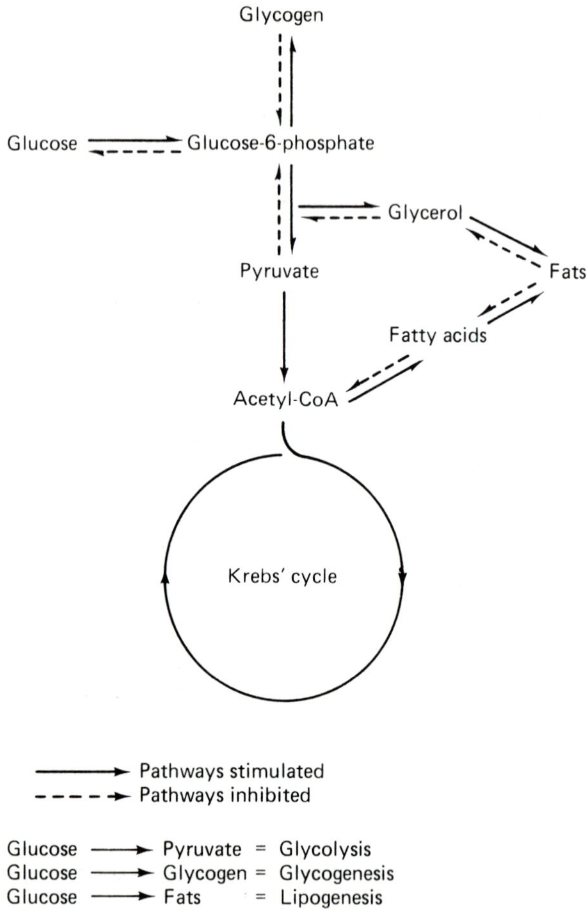

Fig. 1.3 Glucose metabolism after a meal.

glucose. Under aerobic conditions, 1 g of glucose yields energy equivalent to 3.75 kcal or 16 kJ.

2. Excess acetyl-CoA is built up into fatty acids. These combine with glycerol, formed from one of the products of the glycolysis pathway, and are deposited as triglycerides in adipose tissue (lipogenesis).

3. Products of glucose metabolism (in the glycolysis pathway or the Krebs' cycle) are converted to non-essential amino acids (p. 16).

4. Glucose is converted to glycogen for storage in the liver and

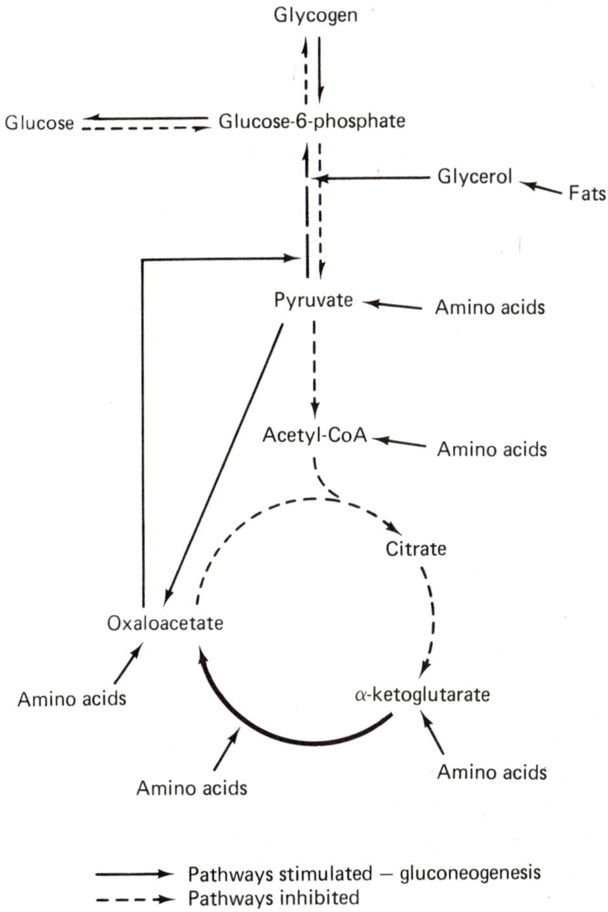

Fig. 1.4 Maintenance of glucose supply.

muscles. The liver contains about 72 g of glycogen (although amounts quoted vary widely). The muscle mass contains some 250 g to 400 g of glycogen, but this is only available for the supply of glucose to the muscle itself.

When an individual is fasting, there are two aspects of metabolism to be considered:

1. The supply of glucose for brain function occurs in two ways (Fig. 1.4):

(a) Breakdown of glycogen to provide glucose.
(b) Gluconeogenesis (formation of new glucose) from glycerol, released when fats are broken down to glycerol and fatty acids, and from amino acids. Amino acids, from protein breakdown, lose the nitrogen-containing portion (deamination) and feed into the Krebs' cycle or glycolysis pathway. The gluconeogenetic pathway is, in essence, the reverse of the glycolysis pathway.

2. The supply of energy for other body tissues is from fat catabolism (*see below*).

FATS (LIPIDS)

These are a heterogeneous group of compounds with the common property of being soluble in organic solvents such as alcohol. They are not soluble in water. A number of different lipids are found in the diet, but can be put into two main groups—simple and compound.

Simple lipids

The simple lipids include the fatty acids and neutral fats. Fatty acids may be saturated or unsaturated. Saturated fatty acids contain the maximum number of hydrogen atoms in combination with the carbon. All the carbon atoms are joined by single bonds.

The general formula is:

$$CH_3(CH_2)_nCOOH$$

Unsaturated fatty acids contain less than the maximum amount of hydrogens and the carbon chain contains at least 1 double bond. The essential fatty acids, which are not made in the body, are polyunsaturated fatty acids with 2 or more double bonds in the carbon chain. These are linoleic (2 double bonds), linoleic (3 double bonds) and arachidonic (4 double bonds) acids.

Neutral fats are formed by the combination of fatty acids with glycerol as mono-, di- or tri-glycerides. These are the major fats in the diet, and the form in which they are stored in adipose tissue.

Glycerol has the structural formula of:

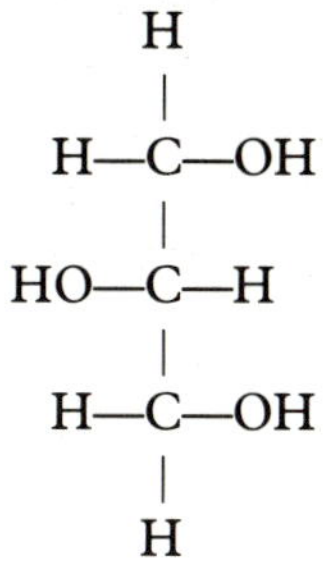

and one fatty acid can combine with each hydroxyl grouping as follows:

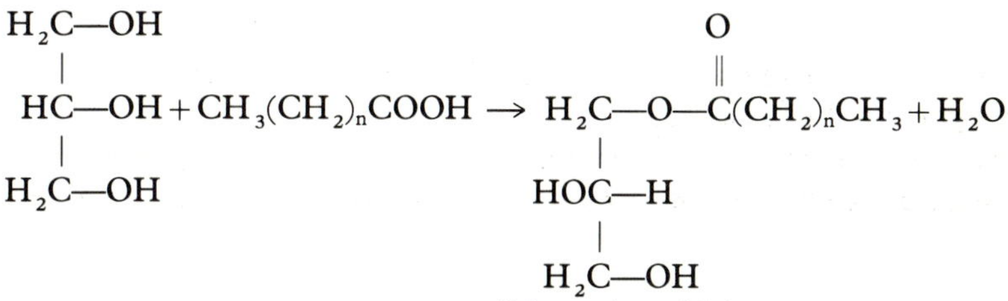

(Monoglyceride)

Compound lipids

This group contains a number of more complex compounds formed from the combination of fatty acids with other substances such as phosphate groups, nitrogenous substances and carbohydrates. It also contains sterols, which are formed around the steroid nucleus, and are the basis for the steroid hormones.

The compound lipids are used as structural fats in the formation of tissue components, the manufacture of hormones and the transport of plasma components.

Neutral fat metabolism

Digestion of fat takes place predominantly in the small intestine by the action of pancreatic lipase, following emulsification by the bile. The end products of fat digestion are:

- Small chain fatty acids.
- Glycerol.
- Large chain fatty acids.
- Partially broken-down triglycerides, i.e. monoglycerides and diglycerides.

The small chain fatty acids and glycerol are absorbed into the portal vein, while the remaining products of digestion are absorbed into the lacteals of the villi and transported into the thoracic duct, eventually emptying into the venous circulation at the junction of the left internal jugular and the left subclavian veins (Fig. 1.5).

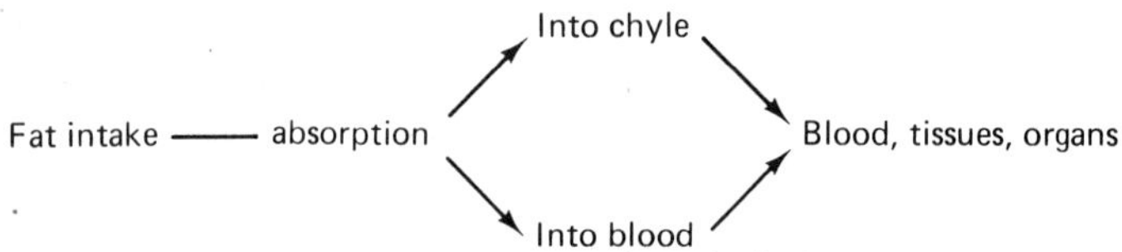

Fig. 1.5 Fat entry into the body.

After absorption, fat is utilized in a number of ways (Fig. 1.6):

1. Fat is stored in the form of triglycerides in the adipose tissue. When necessary (e.g. in fasting) the triglyceride is broken down into glycerol and fatty acids, and used for energy.

2. Fatty acids are catabolized within the mitochondria to acetyl coenzyme-A (Fig. 1.7), which then feeds into the Krebs' cycle (Fig. 1.2). Some ATP is formed during the breakdown to acetyl-CoA, in addition to that formed through the Krebs' cycle. Because of this, fat is a more concentrated source of energy than glucose. The complete breakdown of 1 g of fat to carbon dioxide and water yields 9 kcal (37 kJ).

3. In the liver, fatty acids are broken-down to acetyl-CoA, which is then used to form acetoacetyl-CoA, and then ketones (Fig. 1.7). Ketones are used by most body tissues as an energy source. It is only when these are formed in excessive amounts, as in uncontrolled diabetes mellitus or acute starvation, that they are excreted in quantity in the urine and breath. (Some amino acids can be converted to ketones as an energy source.) Cholesterol, the precursor of steroid hormones, is also formed from acetoacetyl-CoA.

4. The essential fatty acids are thought to be necessary for the formation of prostaglandins—a large group of compounds which have many varied effects within the body. These fatty acids are involved in membrane formation and the normal function of the liver, particularly in lipid transfer.

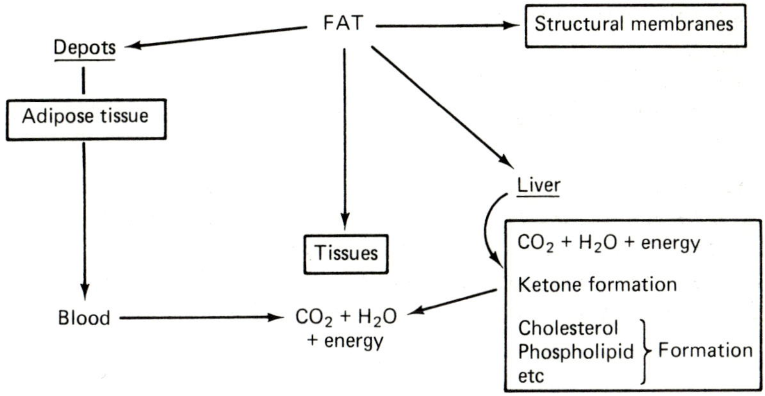

Fig. 1.6 Fat utilization.

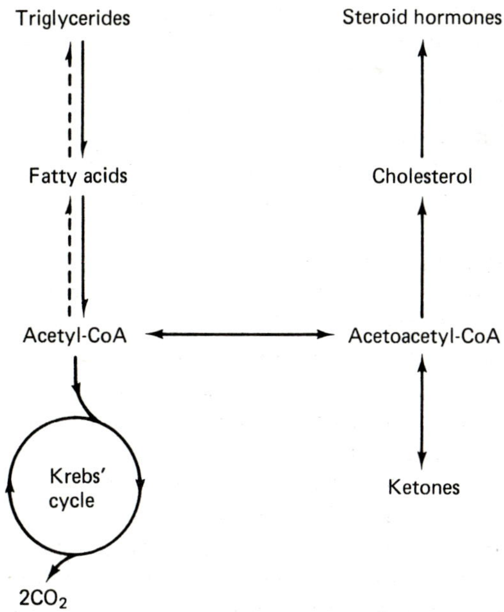

Fig. 1.7 Metabolism of fat.

PROTEINS

Proteins are complex structures of high molecular weight composed of about 20 different amino acids. They are the major constituents of tissues and contain carbon, oxygen, hydrogen and nitrogen with small amounts of other elements such as sulphur. The numerous different proteins in the body are formed by these 20 amino acids in different numbers and combinations.

The diet of most people in the UK contains about 70–100 g of protein a day. The variety of proteins ingested is digested by proteolytic enzymes to amino acids and small peptides. These are absorbed through the intestinal wall into the portal circulation and are transported to the liver. The amino acids are added to the amino acid pool of the body.

Amino acid pool

This refers to the total amount of free amino acid in the blood and the body fluid. It is important to note that there is a constant change in the pool due to a continuous flow of amino acids into and out of it (Fig. 1.8).

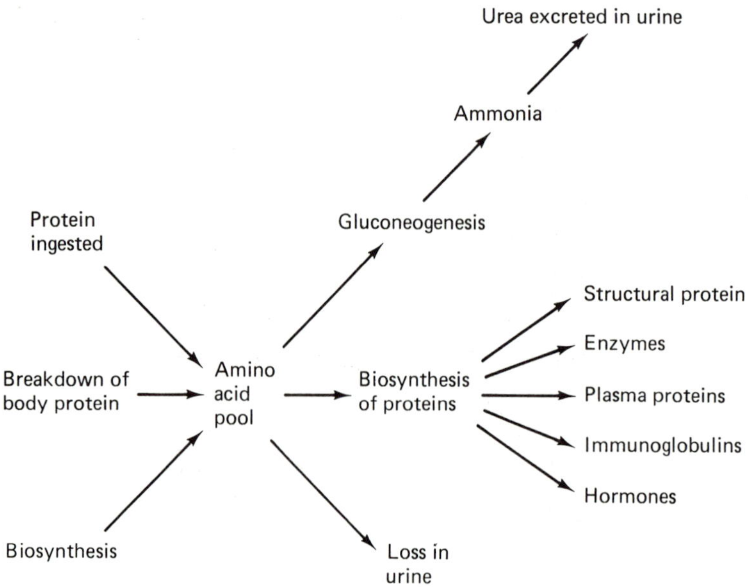

Fig. 1.8 Amino acid metabolism and amino acid pool.

There is a continuous contribution to the pool from the absorption of digested dietary protein, the breakdown of body proteins and the amino acid synthesis in the liver.

Unlike carbohydrates and fats, there is no storage form of amino acids other than the muscle mass of the body. However, the muscle mass is all functional (i.e. it carries out some activity) and, if diminished, the level of activity it sustains is also lessened.

Amino acids are utilized in different ways:

1. The biosynthesis of a number of substances within the body balances the continual catabolism of complex molecules and allows growth and repair of body tissues. Structural proteins within and outside the cell and cellular enzymes are continually being replaced. In addition, the plasma proteins, including immunoglobulins and some hormones, are synthesized from amino acids.

2. As mentioned, amino acids are utilized through gluconeogenesis to form glucose (Fig. 1.4), which is then used for energy by the glucose-dependent tissues. When this is necessary for lengthy periods of time, the muscle mass of the body is reduced. As the protein is used for energy through the formation of glucose, it provides approximately the same amount of energy as glucose (1 g providing 4 kcal/17 kJ). When amino acids are used in this way, the nitrogen-containing part is separated from the rest of the molecule by the process of deamination,

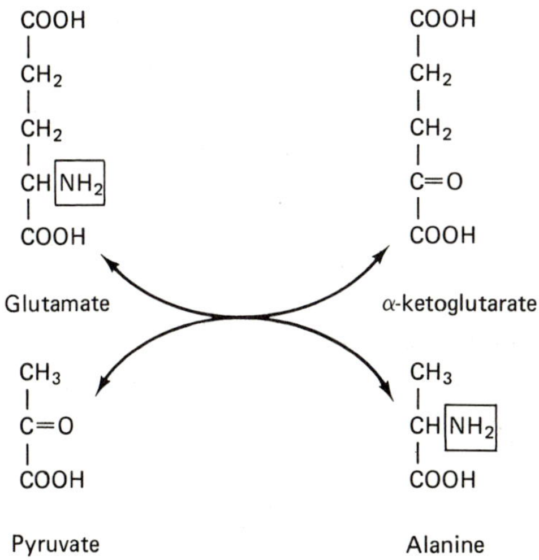

Fig. 1.9 The process of transamination.

which forms ammonia. Ammonia (NH_3) is highly toxic and is converted in the liver to urea, which is harmless, and is excreted in the urine.

3. A number of amino acids are formed within the body as long as a supply of nitrogen is available. The nitrogen required is supplied from other amino acids present in excess. The process is known as transamination, when the amino group is transferred from one molecule to another (Fig. 1.9).

Essential amino acids

While the range of 20 amino acids is essential for growth and replacement of protein tissues, many individual amino acids are synthesized within the body (Fig. 1.9). However, essential amino acids cannot be synthesized, or cannot be formed in adequate amounts within the body. They must, therefore, be included in the diet. The 8 amino acids essential for adults are:

Isoleucine	Methionine	Tryptophan
Leucine	Phenylalanine	Valine
Lysine	Threonine	

Another amino acid, histidine, is also essential for the rapidly growing infant. Arginine may also be required.

INTER-RELATIONSHIP BETWEEN MAJOR NUTRIENTS

The relationship between glucose, fat and amino acid metabolism is illustrated in Fig. 1.10. While there is some degree of interchangeability between them this is limited in extent. Glucose is converted to fat for storage; amino acids are changed to glucose to provide energy. However, for normal body function, adequate glucose must be made available in the diet to prevent excessive breakdown of protein for gluconeogenesis. While fat is a very valuable energy source, it cannot form the glucose essential for brain function. Thus, all the major nutrients must be provided in adequate amounts—including the essential fatty acids and amino acids.

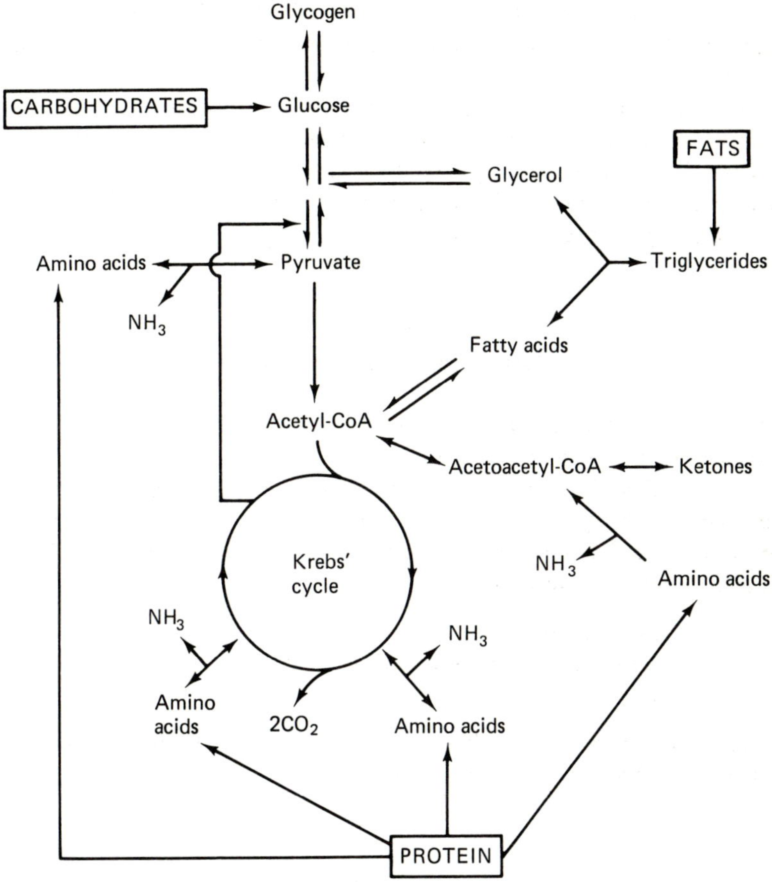

Fig. 1.10 Inter-relationships between major nutrients.

2. Water, Electrolytes and Trace Elements

Before elaborating on body water, electrolytes and the so-called trace elements which make up the body fluid, it is both relevant and useful to describe briefly the concept of the internal environment and the physiology of the body fluid.

Internal environment (milieu intérieur) and homeostasis

Claud Bernard, the French physiologist, introduced the concept of the internal environment by pointing out that the external environment, that is the atmospheric air and all that surrounds us, is not the environment of cells and tissues. Their environment is, in reality, the plasma and the fluid (extracellular fluid) which surrounds and 'baths' them. He referred to this fluid environment as 'the Milieu Intérieur' (the internal environment). He further drew attention to the important fact that, in spite of great variation in the external environment, the composition, pH and temperature of the internal environment is kept fairly constant. That is, there is a state of stability in the environment of the cells without which their lives and functions cannot continue.

The constancy of the internal environment is maintained by numerous complicated physiological and biochemical processes within the body. These readjust the 'climate' of the environment in the face of inevitable change and bring about the necessary stability, which is thus dynamic rather than static.

Maintaining the constancy of the internal environment is a fundamental physiological principle, and is known as homeostasis.

The body has a range of compensatory mechanisms at its disposal to check unacceptable changes which may occur in the composition of this internal environment, and to restore normality. These mechanisms are collectively referred to as homeostatic activities.

BODY WATER

Between 45–70% of body weight is made up of water, that is about 40 l in an individual of 60–70 kg bodyweight. Besides being a good solvent and an excellent carrier for the solutes of the body, water is an essential constituent of all cells and, together with the solutes, make up the internal environment. Water is distributed in all tissues and throughout the body, but the water content of tissues varies in muscles, skin, liver and kidneys. The water content of the body also varies at different stages in life, the elderly containing less than younger people. Due to a larger amount of adipose tissue, women, on average, contain less water than men.

The water is described as being within intracellular and extracellular compartments. The extracellular water occupies the tissue spaces, whereas the intracellular water is contained within the cells of the body. The extracellular compartment is further subdivided into the interstitial compartment surrounding the tissue cells, and the vascular compartment in which the water is accommodated within the blood vessels (plasma-water).

Figure 1.11 and Table 1.1 show the body water distribution into the compartments and their quantitative data.

It is important to appreciate that the division of body water into compartments does not mean complete independence of one compartment from another. There is, in fact, considerable movement of

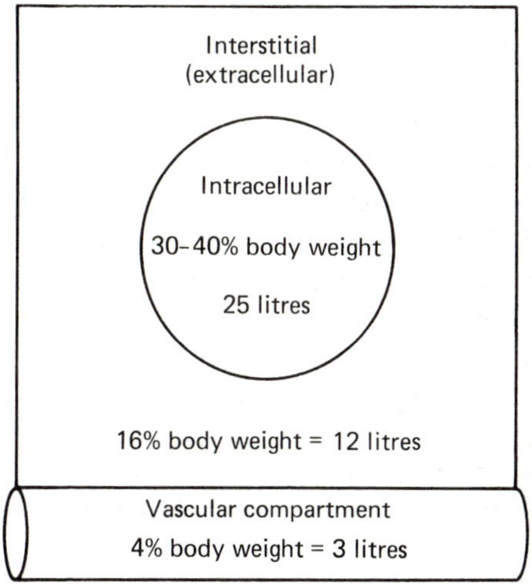

Fig. 1.11 Body water distribution.

Table 1.1 Body water and its distribution

Designation	*Bodyweight* %	*Water* l	*Total body water* %
Total	45–75	40	100
Intracellular	30–40	25	65–70
Interstitial	↗16	↗12	↗20
Extracellular	20	15	30–35
Intravascular	↘4	↘3	↘10

water between the interstitial and vascular compartments on the one hand, and between the extracellular and intracellular compartments on the other. The movement of water between the compartments is governed by pressure gradients (capillary and tissue hydrostatic pressure) and osmosis (crystalloid and 'colloid' osmotic pressures).

Osmosis

The word 'osmosis' is derived from the Greek 'osmos', meaning push, and may be defined as the phenomenon whereby water passes through a semipermeable membrane from a solution of low (very dilute) to one of higher concentration. The effective osmotic pressure is one which, when applied to the more concentrated solution, would prevent water passing through the semipermeable membrane from the solution of lower concentration.

When in contact with a more dilute solution across a semipermeable membrane, the osmotic pressure of a concentrated solution is expressed by the passage of solvent (e.g. water) molecules across the membrane into the more concentrated solution.

The osmotic pressure exerted by a solution is determined by the number of particles in a given volume, and is expressed in osmoles. One osmole (osmol) equals the molecular weight in grams of the substance (1 mol) multiplied by the number of free particles that each molecule liberates in solution. Thus, 1 mol of sodium chloride (NaCl), which liberates 2 ions into solution, would supply 2 osmol, while 1 mol glucose, which does not ionize, will only supply 1 osmol.

The concentration of osmoles is expressed as osmolarity, which is the number of osmoles per litre of solution, or as the osmolality, which is the number of osmoles per kg of solution. One litre of water weighs 1 kg and, in the body, osmotically active substances are dissolved in water so that osmolarity and osmolality are equivalent. The concentration of a solution is expressed in milliosmol/l (i.e. 1/1000 osmol/l) and the osmolality of human plasma is 290 mosm/l (Ganong, 1981).

Solutions exerting similar osmotic pressure to plasma are iso-osmolar (isotonic), while hyperosmolar (hypertonic) solutions have a higher osmolality and hypo-osmolar (hypotonic) solutions have a lower osmolality.

Water turnover and water balance

The maintenance of water balance is among the most important of the body's homeostatic activities. This is achieved through a number of processes, but essentially, over a period of time, the output and intake of water must equal each other in order to maintain normal balance. The intake of water is normally governed by the sensation of thirst and the output is generally controlled by the kidneys. Water is taken by mouth as drinking water and in the fluid content of food. Small amounts of water are made available to the body through metabolism (p. 3). Water is lost principally through the kidneys in the urine and, to a lesser extent, via the skin, lungs (the expired air) and in the faeces. In quantitative terms, some 2500–3000 ml of water is taken into the body during 24 hours. The same amount is also lost by the body so the balance between intake and output is maintained. An example of the amounts gained and lost through different routes during 24 hours is shown in Fig. 1.12. The amounts gained in food, and through its metabolism, are considerable and patients not taking food should be compensated with additional fluid.

This external water balance, or water turnover as it is called, is influenced by, and is part of, a more complex system of internal water

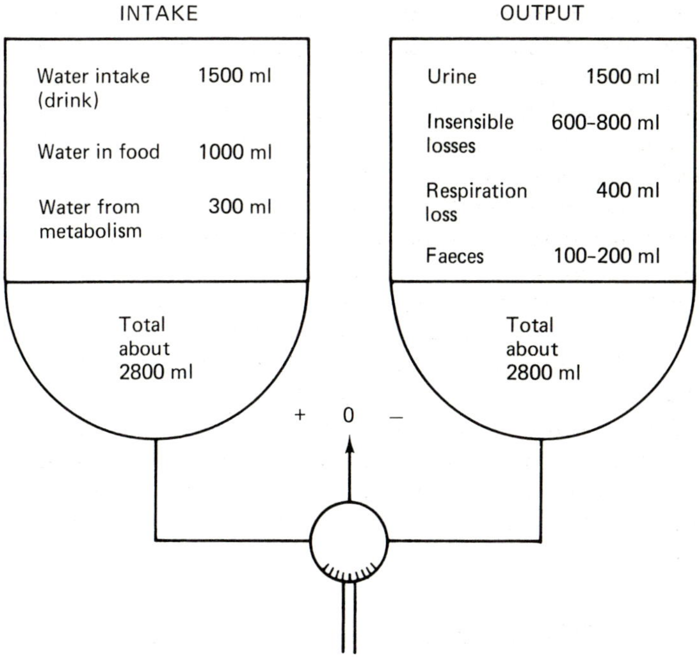

Fig. 1.12 External water turnover.

balance mechanism (internal turnover). The latter is, in the first place, the movement of water between vascular and interstitial compartments (that is across extracellular space), and then between intracellular and extracellular compartments. Whereas the external turnover of water involves 2500–3000 ml/24 h, the internal turnover is concerned with several hundreds of litres of water per day. There is, for instance, a constant exchange of fluid taking place in the alimentary tract through the secretion of saliva and other digestive juices and their subsequent reabsorption. In addition, some 170 l of water per day is filtered through the renal glomeruli and all but about 1500 ml (urinary output) is subsequently reabsorbed by the tubules. Most of all, the exchanges between intracellular and extracellular compartments must amount to several litres per hour.

It is therefore clear that the external water turnover is only a fraction of the total body water turnover, and that the two systems (i.e. external and internal water turnover) are well integrated (Fig. 1.13).

There is, however, a fundamental difference between the mechanisms of water interchange between interstitial and vascular compartments, and the movement of water between intracellular and extracellular fluid compartments. The former is dependent on the physical processes of pressure and osmosis, and takes place freely. The movement of water across the cell membrane to and from the extracellular fluid occurs in response to the distribution of osmotically active particles either side of the cell membrane. This is controlled by active transport of potassium into, and sodium out of, the cell. Considerable amounts of energy are used in pumping sodium and potassium across the cell membrane and, without this, excess sodium and chloride enters the cell, water follows and the cells swell up. The osmolalities of the intracellular and extracellular fluid remain equal due to the activity of the membrane pump.

The interchange of fluid between the vascular and the interstitial fluid compartments takes place at capillary level and is governed by pressure gradients between the compartments.

The factors involved in this fluid exchange (Fig. 1.14; Table 1.2) are as follows:

1. The hydrostatic pressure (i.e. the blood pressure) of capillaries is some 20 mmHg higher at the arterial end (32 mmHg) than at the venous end (12 mmHg). The hydrostatic pressure exerts a force, driving the fluid out of the vascular compartment.

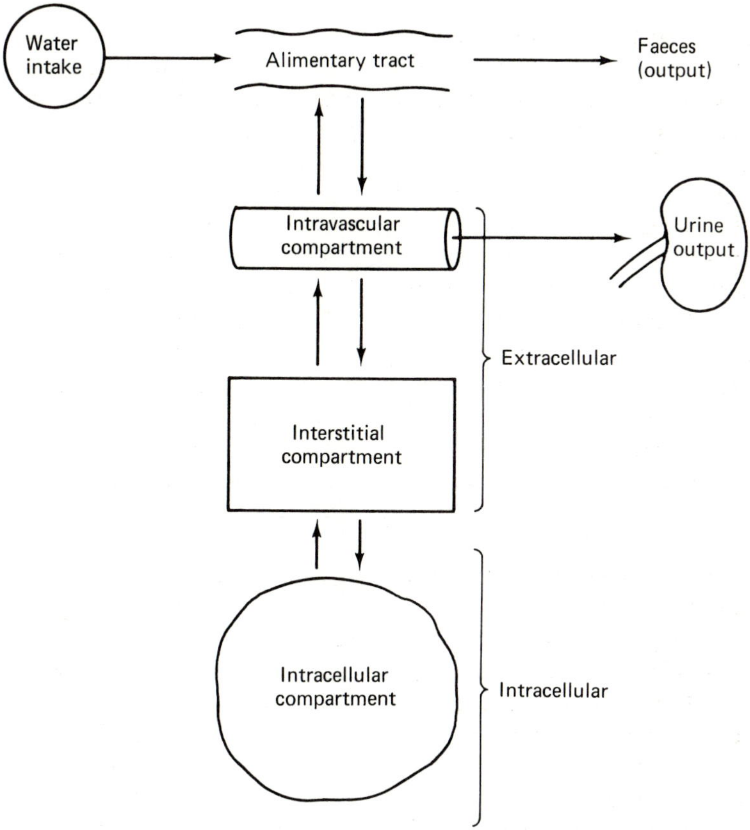

Fig. 1.13 Water turnover.

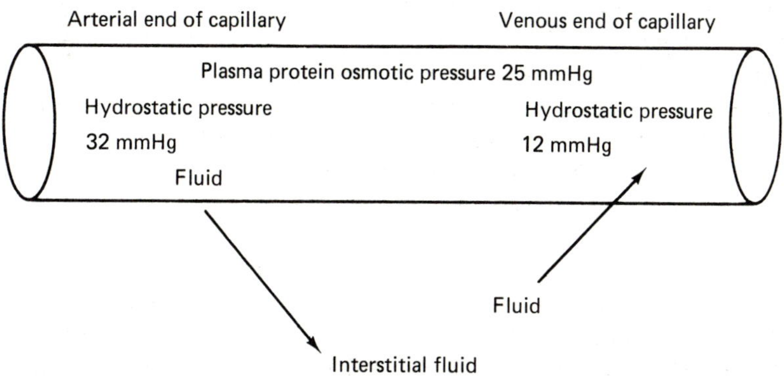

Fig. 1.14 Fluid movement in extracellular space.

Table 1.2 Factors in fluid movement at the capillary

Arterial end	*Venous end*
Outward driving force = 32 mmHg (hydrostatic pressure)	Outward driving force = 12 mmHg (hydrostatic pressure)
Inward driving force = 25 mmHg (plasma protein osmotic pressure)	Inward driving force = 25 mmHg (plasma protein osmotic pressure)
Outward driving force in favour of fluid moving to interstitial compartment } fluid goes out of capillary	Inward driving force in favour of fluid moving to vascular compartment } fluid goes into the capillary
is	is
32 − 25 mmHg = 7 mmHg	25 − 12 mmHg = 13 mmHg

2. The capillaries are surrounded by interstitial (tissue) fluid with a similar pressure at the arterial and the venous ends.

3. The crystalloid osmotic pressure of the vascular compartment (that is of the plasma) exerts an inward force from interstitial to the vascular compartment, but the interstitial fluid has a similar osmotic pressure exerting a force identical to that of the vascular compartment but in the opposite direction (i.e. from the vascular to the interstitial compartment).

4. The vascular compartment contains plasma proteins, which exert an osmotic pressure equal to 25 mmHg. This osmotic pressure (*synonym*: colloid osmotic pressure) exerts an inward force pulling fluid from the interstitial towards the vascular compartment.

The end result of the pressure gradients between the vascular and interstitial compartments is that at the arterial end of the capillary the fluid is driven out of the capillary into the interstitial space, and that at the venous end of the capillary the equivalent amount of fluid re-enters the vascular compartment.

ELECTROLYTES

Many of the substances dissolved in the body water to make up body fluid are found as electrically-charged particles called ions. For instance, the sodium chloride exists in the form of positively charged sodium ions (Na^+) and negatively charged chloride ions (Cl^-). The positively charged ions are *cations*, whereas the negatively charged ones are *anions*. The body fluid ions are called *electrolytes*. In the body fluid, it is the concentration relative to other substances that is important, rather than the total amount of electrolytes present. The unit used to express the concentration of an electrolyte is the 'mole' (mol). The mole is defined as 'the gram-molecular weight of a substance', or the molecular weight in grams of the substance. One mole (mol) of any substance contains approximately 6×10^{23} molecules, thus, by expressing all concentrations in moles/litre (mol/l) a comparison is possible between numbers of particles present. As the amounts found are normally very small, the quantities are divided by 1000 and expressed as millimol/litre (mmol/l).

When the value of an electrolyte in mmol/l is multiplied by its valency, the result is the concentration of the electrolyte in milliequivalents per litre (mEq/l), which is still sometimes seen.

Many of the body fluid electrolytes, such as H^+ (Hydrogen), Na^+ (Sodium), K^+ (Potassium), Cl^- (Chloride) and HCO_3^- (Bicarbonate), have a valency of 1 and therefore their mmol/l = their mEq/l.

Sodium

Sodium is the principal cation of the extracellular fluid, the concentration of which almost equals all anions in the plasma—a total of nearly 3900–4200 mmol. The sodium in the body of an adult is distributed with 40–45% in the skeleton and the remaining distributed through the body fluid. The extracellular fluid contains 140–145 mmol/l whilst the intracellular fluid only has about 15 mmol/l. By its osmotic effect, sodium is an essential element in the body and is particularly concerned with water exchanges within the tissues. The preservation of sodium balance is one of the body's most important homeostatic functions. Daily sodium intake is 80–100 mmol, which is derived from 7–10 g of sodium chloride (common salt) ingested in food. Some 100 mmol of sodium is lost daily from the body, principally in the urine. The basic requirement of sodium is estimated to be 1–1.5 mmol/kg bodyweight/24 h. In catabolic states, and in cases with abnormal losses, 2–3 times this amount is needed to replace the losses and achieve sodium balance.

Potassium

Potassium is the principal cation of the intracellular fluid, where it is found at a concentration of about 157 mmol/l (mEq/l). Plasma and extracellular fluid contains potassium in concentrations of 3.5–5 mmol/l.

The total body potassium is in the order of 2500–3000 mmol, of which nearly 90% is within the cells. Besides its osmotic role within the intracellular compartment, potassium has important functions in neuromuscular transmission, heart and smooth muscle contraction.

The basic daily requirement of potassium is about 1 mmol/kg bodyweight/24 h. In hypercatabolic states, and in cases of abnormal losses, 3–4 times this amount is provided to maintain the balance. As potassium is particularly concentrated within the cells, attention is paid to its provision in the post-injury period, and when tissue protein re-synthesis is taking place.

Calcium

There is a vast reserve of calcium in the body, principally as calcium phosphate and calcium carbonate in the skeleton. Only 1–2% of calcium is distributed in the intracellular and extracellular fluid. Plasma, representing the extracellular fluid, contains 2.1–2.6 mmol/l. (It should be noted that as the valency of Ca^{++} is 2, the plasma concentration is about 5 mEq/l.) The intracellular fluid contains about 1 mmol/l of calcium in ionized form. Half of the plasma calcium is attached to proteins and 50% of plasma calcium is in ionized form. It is the ionized calcium which participates in blood clotting and affects neuromuscular excitability.

The daily requirement of calcium is about 500 mg/day but, because of the large reserve in the skeleton, calcium may not be provided in short-term parenteral feeding.

Magnesium

Like potassium, magnesium is also contained in the cellular compartment. Much of the body magnesium is in the skeleton. Magnesium is necessary for the function of various enzymes concerned with carbohydrate metabolism. The recommended amount in the normal diet is 0.04 mmol/kg/24 h.

OTHER MINERALS AND TRACE ELEMENTS

Besides the elements and electrolytes already described, there are other minerals and elements found in the body that also have important metabolic functions. Many of these are only present in small quantities, but they must nevertheless be provided in the diet. Because of their minute requirements, some are collectively referred to as 'trace elements'. They all participate in enzymatic reactions and act as cofactors in biochemical dissimilations and tissue biosynthesis. The nutritionally important minerals and trace elements are manganese, zinc, copper and phosphorus.

Manganese

This element is concerned with the enzymes involved in carbohydrate metabolism; 0.1 mmol/kg bodyweight/day is estimated as the required amount.

Zinc

Of the total 1.5–2.5 g of zinc in the body, the greater part resides in the skeleton. Plasma zinc level is 1.2–2 mg/l. It is a constituent of a number of cell enzymes and is necessary for wound healing.

The normal diet contains zinc in excess of requirement. The recommended daily amount is about 0.7 mmol/kg/bodyweight. Two important points concerning zinc are:

1. As zinc in the blood is attached to proteins, particularly globulins, its output by the kidneys is increased in cases of proteinuria.
2. Zinc is particularly important in the post-injury period and in tissue repair and, in these circumstances, it should therefore be supplied in a greater amount.

Copper

Some 2 mg (31 mmol) of copper is needed to cover daily requirements. Copper is necessary for the biosynthesis of haemoglobin and incorporation of iron in the porphyrins.

Phosphorus

In addition to its role in ossification, phosphorus is required for many enzymes and participates in metabolic activities of most tissues and energy transfer at tissue level. Patients receiving intravenous nutrition show hypophosphataemia if they are not given an adequate supply. The recommended dose in patients is 10 mmol/day.

Other trace elements

In addition to the above elements, iodine, fluorine, sulphur and cobalt are also necessary for various enzymatic and other metabolic processes.

3. Vitamins

Since the beginning of the century it has been recognized that animals receiving food solely composed of carbohydrates, fats and proteins can not continue to survive, and that other 'accessory food factors' are essential for their living. In man, there are also examples of diseases caused by the lack of these accessory food factors, named 'vitamins' (amines essential to life). There are a variety of vitamins essential for metabolism and, according to their solubility, they are classified as:

- Water soluble (hydrosoluble) vitamins comprising of vitamin B complex and vitamin C.
- Fat soluble (liposoluble) comprising of vitamin A, vitamin D and vitamin K.

HYDROSOLUBLE VITAMINS

Vitamin C (ascorbic acid)

The natural sources of vitamin C are fresh fruits, particularly lemons and oranges, and green vegetables. Its deficiency leads to scurvy, a condition that manifests itself as a haemorrhagic disease, with bleeding tendencies in many sites including gums, joints and skin. Vitamin C is necessary for repair, and affects wound healing.

The daily requirement of vitamin C in the normal diet for an adult is in the order of 25–30 mg.

The recommended allowance in surgical cases varies according to the extent of depletion and requirements for tissue repair.

Vitamin B complex

As the name implies, vitamin B complex comprises a group of water soluble vitamins present in animal tissues. They are related to one another by their actions, which concern carbohydrate and glucose metabolism. Their deficiencies cause conditions such as beri-beri, pellegra and macrocytic anaemia.

Important members of the vitamin B complex are vitamin B_1, B_2, B_3, folic acid and vitamin B_{12}.

Vitamin B_1 (thiamine)

The natural sources of vitamin B_1 are cereals and yeasts. Deficiency of this vitamin leads to beri-beri, which is a carbohydrate metabolic disorder affecting the nervous and cardiovascular systems.

The daily recommended requirement of thiamine in an adult is 0.7–1.2 mg, according to the level of metabolic activities. Females require less than males of the same age and level of metabolism.

Vitamin B_2 (riboflavin)

The natural sources of vitamin B_2 are meat and wholemeal flour. Its deficiency leads to stomatitis and dermatitis. The daily requirement for an adult is 1.2–1.7 mg.

Vitamin B_3 (nicotinic acid)

This vitamin is also known as vitamin PP. The natural sources of vitamin B_3 are liver, kidney and yeasts, and it forms the active molecule of co-enzymes involved in carbohydrate metabolism. Deficiency of this vitamin is responsible for the development of pellegra, characterized by asthenia, anorexia and cutaneous lesions. The estimated daily requirement for an adult is about 15–18 mg.

Folic acid

Folic acid is a member of the vitamin B complex group and is found in animal tissues such as liver, kidney and muscles. Its deficiency is responsible for abnormalities of cell division, anaemia of megaloblastic variety and neurological disorders. Its daily requirement is 10–30 mg.

Vitamin B_{12} (cyanocobalamin)

This vitamin is synthesized entirely by micro-organisms and is stored in the liver. In man, the intestinal synthesis cannot fully cover the requirements. The action of vitamin B_{12} is intimately related to that of folic acid and a deficiency leads to macrocytic anaemia and neuropathy (subacute combined degeneration of the spinal cord). The daily requirement for an adult is about 3 mg obtained from animal products, particularly liver.

LIPOSOLUBLE VITAMINS

Vitamin A

In ordinary food, vitamin A is found in the fat of milk and some green vegetables and carrots. Its deficiency causes salivary and lacrimal gland atrophy, with consequent dryness of mouth and xerophthalmia (dryness of eye). Vitamin A's action on visual purple is noteworthy in that its deficiency can lead to night blindness.

The daily requirement of vitamin A is around 700–750 μg.

Vitamin D

Vitamin D is found in milk, fish and liver and is formed in the skin when exposed to sunlight. Its deficiency in children leads to rickets, with decalcification and consequent softening of the bones. In adults, the same deficiency causes osteomalacia.

The recommended requirement of vitamin D for an adult is about 2.5 μg/day; children require much more (about 10 μg/day).

Vitamin K

The natural sources of vitamin K are green vegetables. This vitamin is necessary for the synthesis of prothrombin, an essential clotting factor. Its deficiency leads to disorders of blood coagulation.

The daily requirement of vitamin K is not precisely determined, but for an adult on a normal diet 2 mg/day is recommended.

4. Nutrition and Diet in Health

The utilization of nutrients by the body cells is discussed on p. 3. However, to plan the nutritional intake for a patient, it is necessary to know the amounts of nutrients required in health and to consider their modification during illness or after surgery.

NUTRIENT INTAKE

Protein, carbohydrate and fat are required by the body in amounts sufficient for the provision of enough energy to fuel all the body's activities, and to supply substances needed for replacement of body tissues. A balance between the amount of energy and the protein in the diet is needed. If an adequate source of energy is not taken in the diet, then protein is broken down for this purpose and the nitrogen in the protein excreted. The individual is then in a state of negative nitrogen balance. Clearly, the amounts of nutrients needed vary according to age and size, to physiological state (growth, pregnancy, lactation) and to the amount of activity undertaken. The Department of Health and Social Security (DHSS) have prepared a recommended daily intake of nutrients (Table 1.3), which gives the amount of nutrient (including some vitamins and minerals) recommended to supply the needs of the majority of healthy people. It therefore follows that some people ingesting the amounts suggested will receive more than is necessary. (The amounts of energy recommended are based on the average needs of persons in the UK.)

Table 1.3 is only a guide to the needs of a particular individual, as people vary in their requirements which, in addition, may be reduced due to inactivity, or increased due to the illness or trauma.

Essential amino acids must be present in the diet in adequate amounts. If not, other amino acids cannot be utilized to form body protein and are subsequently metabolized.

Animal protein contains all the necessary amino acids and is therefore a valuable protein source. In a vegetarian diet, however, it is possible to ingest a satisfactory mix of amino acids by the judicious combination of foods at each meal.

Similarly, essential fatty acids must be included. The best source for these is vegetable oils used in cooking. There is some evidence that an increased use of oils, and a corresponding decrease in the use of animal fat in the diet, may give some protection against the development of atherosclerosis.

In addition to energy and protein, a complete diet must also supply adequate amounts of water, minerals and vitamins.

TYPE OF DIET

The nutrients required are supplied in the diet in an almost infinite variety of combinations and forms of preparation. A diet containing a good variety of foodstuffs is likely to provide adequate amounts of all the different nutrients, assuming of course that adequate amounts of food are ingested and nutrients have not been destroyed in the food's preparation. For example, water soluble vitamins are lost into the water during cooking and vitamin C, in particular, is destroyed by air or cooking.

The *Manual of Nutrition*, published by the Ministry of Agriculture, Fisheries and Food (1976), is a useful guide to the nutrient content of various foods and the effects of preparation.

Though many different types of diet still provide adequate nutrients for health, it is important to find out from patients what types of foods they eat and in what quantities, so that possible deficiencies may be identified. Those who eat little fruit and vegetables may be on the borderline of vitamin C deficiency. The elderly tend to have difficulty eating fresh fruit, and are therefore more likely to have a subclinical deficiency of Vitamin C. Vegetarians, particularly Vegans who eat no animal products at all, are at risk of a deficiency of vitamin B_{12}. Asian women, who by their clothing are exposed to little sunlight and who may eat little margarine, milk or fish, may be short of vitamin D. If such possible deficiencies are identified before overt signs develop, then adequate nutritional supplements can be given.

One item in the diet not yet mentioned is fibre. This is not utilized by the body cells and its value lies in the effect of its presence on the absorption of other nutrients, and in the elimination of waste from the gut. Fibre is the indigestible remains of food ingested and is mainly the residue from fruit and vegetables, whole grain cereals and bread. It is suggested that, when carbohydrate is eaten in the form of high fibre foods, the glucose from digestion is made available to the body more slowly. Therefore, the blood glucose level will rise more slowly after a meal, and the insulin secreted is less (Reaven *et al.*, 1979). Fibre adds bulk to the gut contents, and movement of waste material through the bowel is facilitated. Bowel function therefore tends to be more frequent and the consistency of the stools is softer.

STAGES IN LIFE CYCLE

While the same nutrients are required at different stages in life, the specific requirements may vary. During growth, the healthy child is in positive nitrogen balance as additional muscle is being laid down in

Table 1.3 Recommended daily intakes of energy and nutrients for the UK, 1969 (Department of Health and Social Security)

Age range[a] in years	*Occupational category*	*Bodyweight[c]*	*Energy[d]*		*Protein[f]*	*Thiamin[g]*	*Riboflavin*	*Nicotinic Acid*	*Ascorbic Acid*	*Vitamin A*	*Vitamin D[j]*	*Calcium*	*Iron*
		kg	kcal	MJ[e]	g	mg	mg	mg equiv[h]	mg	μg retinol equiv[i]	μg chole-calci-ferol	mg	mg
Boys and girls													
0 up to 1[b]	—	7.3	800	3.3	20	0.3	0.4	5	15	450	10.0	600[l]	6[l]
1 up to 2	—	11.4	1200	5.0	20	0.5	0.6	7	20	300	10.0	500	7
2 up to 3	—	13.5	1400	5.9	35	0.6	0.7	8	20	300	10.0	500	7
3 up to 5	—	16.5	1600	6.7	40	0.6	0.8	9	20	300	10.0	500	8
5 up to 7	—	20.5	1800	7.5	45	0.7	0.9	10	20	300	2.5	500	8
7 up to 9	—	25.1	2100	8.8	53	0.8	1.0	11	20	400	2.5	500	10
Boys													
9 up to 12	—	31.9	2500	10.5	63	1.0	1.2	14	25	575	2.5	700	13
12 up to 15	—	45.5	2800	11.7	70	1.1	1.4	16	25	725	2.5	700	14
15 up to 18	—	61.0	3000	12.6	75	1.2	1.7	19	30	750	2.5	600	15

Girls													
9 up to 12	—	33.0	2300	9.6	58	0.9	1.2	13	25	575	2.5	700	13
12 up to 15	—	48.6	2300	9.6	58	0.9	1.4	16	25	725	2.5	700	14
15 up to 18	—	56.1	2300	9.6	58	0.9	1.4	16	30	750	2.5	600	15
Men													
18 up to 35	Sedentary	65.0	2700	11.3	68	1.1	1.7	18	30	750	2.5	500	10
	Moderately active	—	3000	12.6	75	1.2	1.7	18	30	750	2.5	500	10
	Very active	—	3600	15.1	90	1.4	1.7	18	30	750	2.5	500	10
35 up to 65	Sedentary	65.0	2600	10.9	65	1.0	1.7	18	30	750	2.5	500	10
	Moderately active	—	2900	12.1	73	1.2	1.7	18	30	750	2.5	500	10
	Very active	—	3600	15.1	90	1.4	1.7	18	30	750	2.5	500	10
65 up to 75	Assuming a sedentary	63.0	2350	9.8	59	0.9	1.7	18	30	750	2.5	500	10
75 and over	life	63.0	2100	8.8	55	0.8	1.7	18	30	750	2.5	500	10
Women													
18 up to 55	Most occupations	55.0	2200	9.2	55	0.9	1.3	15	30	750	2.5	500	12
	Very active	—	2500	10.5	63	1.0	1.3	15	30	750	2.5	500	12
55 up to 75	Assuming a seden-	53.0	2050	8.6	51	0.8	1.3	15	30	750	2.5	500	10
75 and over	tary life	53.0	1900	8.0	48	0.7	1.3	15	30	750	2.5	500	10
Pregnancy, 2nd and 3rd trimester	—	—	2400	10.0	60	1.0	1.6	18	60	750	10.0[k]	1200[m]	15
Lactation	—	—	2700	11.3	68	1.1	1.8	21	60	1200	10.0	1200	15

Footnotes on next page

a The ages are from one birthday to another: e.g., 9 up to 12 is from the 9th up to, but not including, the 12th birthday. The figures in the Table in general refer to the mid-point ranges, though those for the range 18 up to 35 refer to the age 25 years, and for the range 18 up to 55, to 35 years of age.

b Average figures relating to the first year of life.

c The bodyweights of children and adolescents are averages and relate to London in 1965 (Tanner, Whitehouse and Takaishi, 1966). The bodyweights of adults do not represent average values; they are those of the FAO (1957*a*) reference man and woman, with a nominal reduction for the elderly.

d Average requirements relating to groups of individuals.

e Megajoules (10^6 J). Calculated from the relation 1 kcal = 4.186 kJ, and rounded to 1 decimal place.

f Recommended intakes calculated as providing 10% of energy requirements.

g The figures, calculated from energy requirements and the recommended intake of thiamin of 0.4 mg/1000 kcal, relate to groups of individuals.

h 1 nicotinic acid equivalent = 1 mg available nicotinic acid or 60 mg tryptophan.

i 1 retinol equivalent = 1 µg retinol or 6 µg β-carotene or 12 µg other biologically active carotenoids.

j No dietary source may be necessary for those adequately exposed to sunlight, but the requirement for the housebound may be greater than that recommended.

k For all three trimesters.

l These figures apply to infants who are not breast fed. Infants who are entirely breast fed receive smaller quantities; these are adequate since absorption from breast milk is higher.

m For the third trimester only.

the body and the proportion of protein needed is greater. The diet must therefore include all the essential amino acids (including histidine and possibly arginine). Energy requirements are also high in relation to weight, and minerals and vitamins must be supplied in adequate amounts during this period to maintain normal growth and development.

During adult life, the body is in a state of equilibrium. The amount of nitrogen ingested in protein is equal to the amount lost in urea and other waste products. The individual is in nitrogen balance and protein is only needed in amounts large enough to balance the protein breakdown during the normal turnover of tissue constituents.

During pregnancy and lactation, a woman naturally has an increased requirement for virtually all nutrients (Table 1.3).

The elderly, who form a large proportion of hospital patients, even on general wards, require the same nutrients as others but, as their activity decreases, will need a lower energy intake. Because of economic difficulties and problems in mobility, leading to difficulty in shopping and food preparation, the elderly may have an inadequate diet. This may lead to nutritional deficiencies, which will become obvious when they are put under any additional stress (e.g. by illness or operation).

5. Metabolism in Starvation

When the diet is deficient in energy and protein, essential metabolic requirements have to be met by the body stores.

The carbohydrate (as glycogen) and fat stores, and body protein, can all be used for energy (p. 5). The glycogen store in the liver and muscles is about 327 g (in a 70 kg man), but only about 72 g of glycogen in the liver is available for maintenance of blood glucose, and will only last a short time (Ganong, 1981). The blood glucose level is also maintained by gluconeogenesis from amino acids and the glycerol of fats. However, glycerol plays only a small part in the supply of glucose.

In starvation, many tissues of the body use ketones and fatty acids, in preference to glucose, as an energy source. Initially the brain is dependent on glucose, and deamination of amino acids for gluconeogenesis is essential. However, over a period of about 4–5 days, the brain cells produce the enzymes required to metabolize ketones for energy. This adaptive facility of the brain helps to preserve the protein content of the body, as gluconeogenesis from amino acids becomes less important. Fat becomes the major energy source for the body cells, as both fatty acids and ketones are utilized.

However, amino acids are required for the replacement of protein broken down as a normal part of body metabolism. All body proteins, including cell enzymes, have a limited life and are normally replaced in equilibrium with destruction. Nevertheless, without adequate essential amino acids and an adequate nitrogen source, this cannot occur and muscle wasting develops. The individual goes into a state of negative nitrogen balance as the amino acids, which cannot be used for protein synthesis, are deaminated and the nitrogen excreted as urea.

During starvation the metabolic rate falls to enable the body stores to last as long as possible. The glycogen stores of the body last only short periods of time before fat and protein breakdown occurs. Fat catabolism leads to excessive formation of ketones, some of which will be excreted via the lungs and in the urine, but does not usually lead to acidosis. Protein breakdown and loss results in a reduction in muscle mass and strength and eventually the levels of plasma proteins fall, leading to oedema. Blood glucose levels are maintained for as long as possible.

Loss of body weight occurs slowly in uncomplicated starvation, and death occurs when 40–50% of weight is lost.

Many patients, who require artificial feeding, exhibit some of the metabolic changes associated with starvation.

6. Metabolic Response in Trauma and Injury

For over 50 years it has been recognized that following trauma, including a surgical operation, there is an immediate but temporary metabolic change within the body, the duration of which is related to the severity and extent of the injury. The physiological rationale of these metabolic alterations is best understood by observing injured animals.

After injury, the animal is not able to hunt or search for food and has to rely on body fluid and stores of nutrients. Besides the basic nutritional requirements, the animal is also in need of materials for repair and healing processes which have to receive priority for nutrients over some of the less vital parts of the body. Therefore, on the one hand, the body's economy demands the preservation of fluid and the usage of stored energy and proteins, while on the other, the diversion of resources to the needy area is required.

One aspect of the metabolic response to injury is that of water and sodium conservation. This phenomenon is vital as the sodium ion is the most important electrolyte for the preservation of the internal environment ('milieu intérieur' of Claud Bernard, p. 18) and its conservation after injury is a logical step by the body to preserve the constancy, including the volume, of that environment. The energy requirements at this time are derived from the body reserves of carbohydrate, fat and protein. The latter, in effect, form a major source of energy after injury because of the limited quantity of the carbohydrate store and the necessity of maintaining the blood glucose level after trauma. Proteins are broken down (catabolized) and release amino acids which in turn, following deamination, become a source of energy. The nitrogen residue of these amino acids is then excreted in the urine as urea and accounts for the increase in urinary nitrogen excretion immediately following injury. Protein catabolism also releases numerous essential and non-essential amino acids needed for repair and wound healing.

Observations made on patients after trauma, or surgical operation, have found behavioural and metabolic changes similar to those in animals. After surgical operations, for instance, the patient lies quietly and usually likes to remain undisturbed and normally shows no interest in eating. Metabolic and biochemical studies of such individuals show a reduction in water and sodium excretion, and an increase in urinary excretion of nitrogen, potassium and phosphorus.

The immediate post-traumatic period, in which there is altered metabolism characterized by protein breakdown resulting in excess nitrogen loss and negative nitrogen balance, is referred to as the catabolic phase of injury. During this early post-traumatic or post-operative phase, the catabolic process results in loss of muscle mass, with subsequent increase in nitrogen loss in the urine (Fig. 1.15), and a general reduction in bodyweight.

The original work of Cuthbertson in the 1930s, and that of many others since, has established that the duration and severity of the

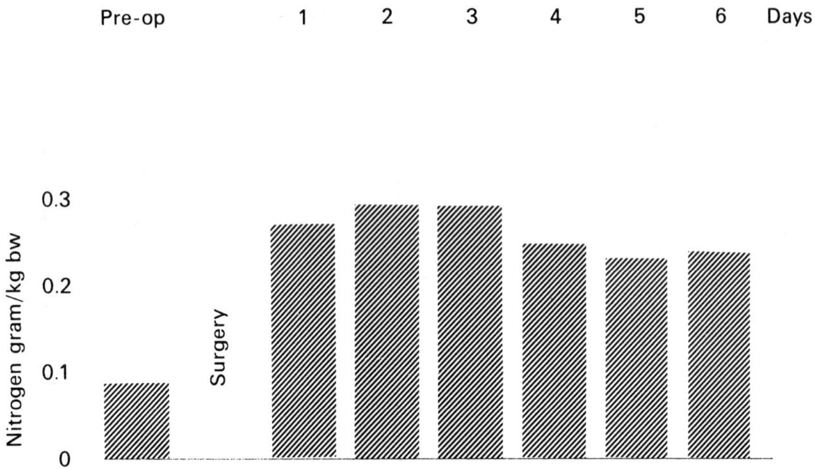

Fig. 1.15 Mean nitrogen excretion in 5 patients after surgery. It can be seen that pre-operatively the mean nitrogen loss has been 0.09 g/kg bodyweight; the first 3 days after operation has raised the nitrogen loss to over three times the pre-operative level 0.27 to 0.29 g/kg bodyweight and, on days 4, 5 and 6, a gradual reduction has taken place.

catabolic phase of the post-traumatic or post-surgical metabolic changes is related to the extent and severity of the injury—the response to a fracture of femur, appendicectomy and oesophagectomy will vary in degree of severity.

After a time the catabolic phase of an injury is followed by an anabolic phase, during which food is used to build up structural proteins. This leads to retention of nitrogen, reduced nitrogen excretion and results in a positive nitrogen balance. In this recovery phase the patient gains weight as the muscle mass increases, and begins to regain interest in work and other activities.

The mechanisms underlying the metabolic response to injury and surgery have been studied in some depth. It is clear that the changes which occur are similar to those in the stress response, which develop as a result of numerous types of stressor, including psychological factors such as anxiety. In all these situations there is an alteration in activity of the hypothalamus and (partly through the action of hypothalamic hormones which modulate its activity) of the pituitary and adrenal glands. The regulatory role of the hypothalamus on the endocrine system is shown in Fig. 1.16, and indicates that in times of stress

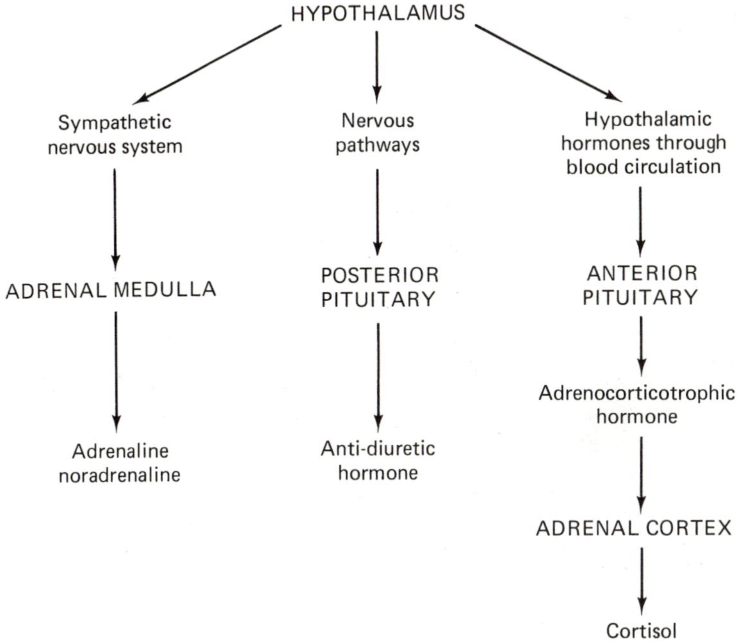

Fig. 1.16 The role of the hypothalamus in stress.

(whatever the cause) the changes in the endocrine system may be widespread. However, the metabolic changes following trauma and surgery are mainly due to an increase in the secretion of antidiuretic hormone from the posterior pituitary gland, and of adrenocorticotrophic hormone from the anterior pituitary gland, which then stimulates the release of adrenocorticosteroid hormones, particularly cortisol.

The glucocorticoid hormones, of which cortisol is one, are mainly responsible for the catabolic changes which occur. In excess, the catabolic effects of these hormones may be harmful (e.g. wound healing is reduced, or the immune response lowered). However the ability to respond to stress, by an increase in the secretion of these hormones, is essential for adaptation and normal recovery from surgery or trauma. Nevertheless, as some effects may be harmful, it is important that the stress response is modified by reducing anxiety through effective communication, i.e. giving accurate information, clarifying misconceptions, etc. (Boore, 1978).

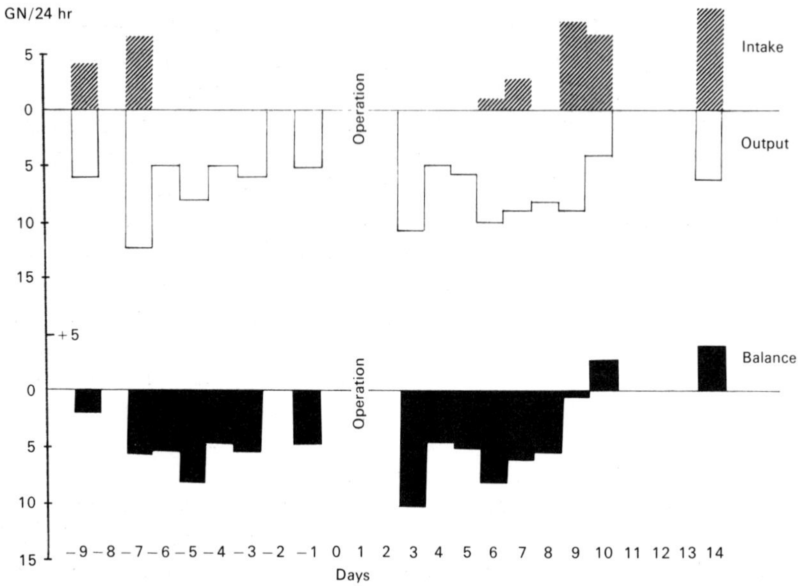
GN/24 hr
Intake
Output
Operation
Balance
Operation
+5
Days

(a)

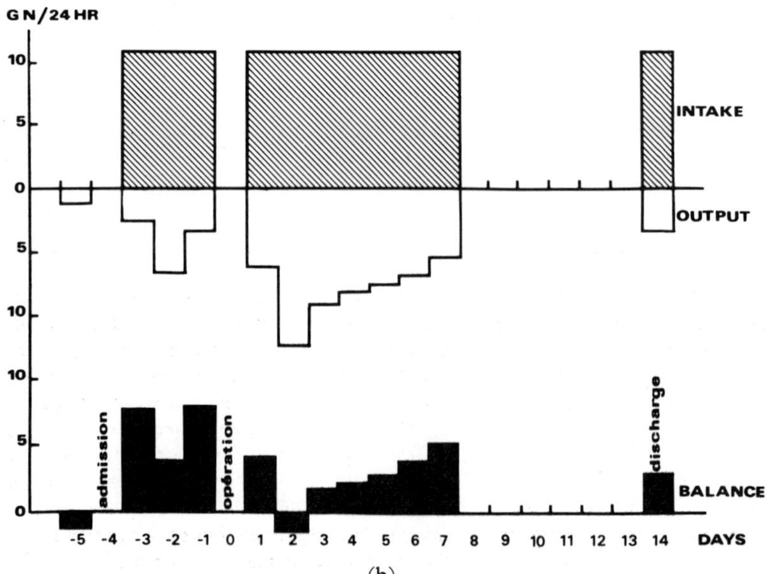
GN/24 HR
INTAKE
OUTPUT
admission
operation
discharge
BALANCE
DAYS

(b)

Knowledge of the metabolic response to injury has important practical implications. For instance, a number of workers have shown that the post-traumatic catabolic phase can be shortened, and the negative nitrogen balance checked, if a high protein and calorie intake is provided (Figs 1.17a,b). It also seems that the therapeutic reversal of nitrogen balance from negative to positive has beneficial effects on the clinical progress of patients, and is attended by a more favourable prognosis. In addition, after surgery, the fluid retention in the body is increased by ADH secretion and the administration of an extra volume of i.v. fluid to patients may not improve output, but can lead to fluid overload and give rise to pulmonary and cerebral symptoms. When intravenous fluid is infused postoperatively, careful monitoring of the patient's clinical condition and biochemical profile is essential because, at that time, the patient's homeostatic activities with regard to water and electrolyte balance are impaired.

After extensive trauma, the body reserves of energy and protein may be affected to such an extent as to deplete the body of the essential protein constituents necessary for enzymatic activities at cellular level, with consequent impairment of function leading to deterioration in the state of health. It is this context that gives the basis for the rationale of postoperative artificial nutrition (be it parenteral or enteral), and it is for this reason that the greater the trauma, and more extensive the catabolism, the higher level of nutritional support necessary.

Fig. 1.17 (a) Nitrogen balance of a patient not receiving artificial feeding before and after major surgery. The patient was suffering from cancer of the oesophagus and was given intravenous fluid and electrolytes before and immediately after the operation. The upper portion of the graph indicates nitrogen intake and output in g/24 hours, and the lower portion shows clearly the negative nitrogen balance until the patient was able to resume normal food intake. (b) Nitrogen balance of a patient receiving artificial feeding before and after major surgery. The patient was suffering from cancer of the oesophagus and was given parenteral nutrition with high energy and nitrogen levels before and immediately after operation (to day 7). The upper portion of the graph shows nitrogen intake and output and the lower portion shows the generally positive nitrogen balance.

REFERENCES

Bernard C. (1885). *Lecon sur les phenomenes de la vie communes aux animaux et aux vegeteaux*. Paris: Balliere.

Boore J.R.P. (1978). *Prescription for Recovery*. London: Royal College of Nursing.

Cuthbertson D.P. (1930). The disturbance of metabolism produced by bony and non-bony injury with notes on certain abnormal conditions of bones. *Biochemical Journal*; **24**: 1244–1263.

Cuthbertson D.P. (1932). Observation on the disturbance of metabolism produced by injury to limbs. *Quarterly Journal of Medicine*; **25**: 333–346.

Ganong W.F. (1981). *Review of Medical Physiology*. 10th edn. Los Altos, California: Lange Medical Publications.

Martin D.W., Mayes P.A., Rodwell V.W. (1981). *Harper's Review of Biochemistry*. 18th edn. Los Altos, California: Lange Medical Publications.

Ministry of Agriculture, Fisheries and Food (1976). *Manual of Nutrition*. London: HMSO.

Reaven G.M., Coulston A.M., Marcus A.M. (1979). Nutritional management of diabetes. Symposium on Applied Nutrition in Clinical Medicine. *The Medical Clinics of North America*; **63**(5): 927–943.

Tanner J.M., Whitehouse R.H., Takaishi M. (1966). Standards from birth to maturity for height, weight, height velocity and weight velocity: British children. *Arch Dis. Child*; **41**: 454–471.

FURTHER READING

Burch R.E., Hahn M.K.J. (1979). Trace elements in human nutrition. *The Medical Clinics of North America*; **63**(5): 1057–1068.

Cox T. (1978). *Stress*. London: Macmillan.

Davidson S., Passmore R., Brock J.F., Truswell A.S. (1975). *Human Nutrition and Dietetics*. 6th edn. Edinburgh: Churchill Livingstone.

Dickerson J.W.T., Lee H.A. (1978). *Nutrition in the Clinical Management of Disease*. London: Edward Arnold.

Golden M.N.H., Golden B.E. (1981). Trace elements: potential importance in human nutrition with particular reference to zinc and vanadium. *British Medical Bulletin*; **37**: 31–36.

Huskisson J.M. (1981). *Nutrition and Dietetics in Health and Disease*. London: Balliere Tindall.

Jeejeebhoy K.N. (1981). Protein nutrition in clinical practice. *British Medical Bulletin*; **37**: 11–17.

Krause M.V., Mahan L.K. (1979). *Food, Nutrition and Diet Therapy*. 6th edn. Philadelphia: W.B. Saunders.

Moore F.D. (1959). Metabolism in trauma: the reaction of survival. Symposium on Metabolism after Trauma. *Metabolism*; 8.

Moore F.D., Ball M.R. (1952). *The Metabolic Response to Surgery*. Springfield, Illinois: Charles C. Thomas.

Richards J.R. (1980). Current concepts in the metabolic responses to injury,

infection and starvation. *Proceedings of the Nutritional Society*; **39**: 113–123.
Selye M. (1956). *The Stress of Life*. New York: McGraw-Hill Book Co.
Symposium on Surgical Nutrition (1981). *The Surgical Clinics of North America*; **61**(3).
Underwood E.J. (1981). Trace elements in human and animal health. *Journal of Human Nutrition*; **35**: 37–48.
Waterlow J.C., Jackson A.A. (1981). Nutrition and protein turnover in man. *British Medical Bulletin*; **37**: 5–10.

SECTION II

Artificial Feeding

This section considers the development of artificial feeding and discusses, in detail, nutritional assessment. This is the first stage in the nutritional management of any patient, and sets the scene for Sections III and IV where different modes of artificial feeding are considered. Patients receiving artificial feeding, irrespective of the method used, have many nursing needs and the care of these patients is outlined. The care related to the specific method of nutritional support is discussed in Sections III, IV.

7. Development of Clinical Nutrition and Artificial Feeding

Eating is not only one of the pleasures of life but is also the most agreeable, desirable and physiological way of providing nutrients to the body. There are, however, circumstances in which food cannot be ingested, digested or absorbed, and the nutrients do not therefore reach their destination—the metabolic pool of the body. In these circumstances, artificial nutrition becomes necessary to support metabolism.

The idea of artificial feeding and nutritional support is not a new one. In the words of Sir David Cuthbertson (1980): 'Down through the ages all who have had to tend the gravely injured or patients who by the nature of their operation or medical defect have been unable to ingest, digest or absorb an adequate supply of nutrients, have been greatly concerned and, until relatively recently, frustrated in having to solve the problems'.

The need for artificial feeding in these patients is now fully recognized, but methods and suitable nutrients have only been clinically exploited in the 20th century when artificial feeding has become a reality. It is now possible to provide support for a variety of patients who cannot otherwise be nutritionally and metabolically self-sufficient. Some patients with an acute metabolic crisis are dramatically helped to their recovery. Others with partial or total alimentary tract failure are supported partially or totally by artificial feeding.

One of the less spectacular, but none the less important, recent developments in artificial feeding and clinical nutrition as a whole is an awareness by doctors, nurses and all involved in the day-to-day management of patients of the importance of nutrition. Paradoxically, however, it is possible to discover malnutrition developing in some hospital patients under the very eyes of those who treat the disease and not the patients. There is no justification for patients to starve due to repeated periods of 'nil by mouth' for clinical investigations. These should be recorded and compensated. With methods of feeding, and a range of nutrient solutions available for use, it is a sad indictment that a patient's nutritional status can be seen to decline while they are receiving hospital care. It has been said that a hospital is the only place where people can legally be starved!

ARTIFICIAL FEEDING

Artificial nutrition may be defined as the provision of made-up food (i.e. feeds containing the required nutrients for an artificial feeding regime that are prepared within the hospital) or chemically-defined, manufactured nutrients to the body, through an artificial system of administration. The routes used are the alimentary tract in enteral feeding, or some other route, usually intravenous, in parenteral feeding.

Parenteral feeding

The term 'parenteral feeding' (intravenous feeding/parenteral nutrition) refers to a method of supplying nutrients by means other than that of the alimentary tract. In practice, this means the administration of nutrient solutions into the venous system of the circulation. Parenteral nutrition is now synonymous with intravenous feeding (IVF) and when nutrition is entirely undertaken by parenteral methods alone, the term 'total parenteral nutrition' (TPN) is applied. When nutrition is partially supported by parenteral feeding, the term 'supplementary parenteral feeding', or 'supplementary parenteral nutrition' (SPN) is used.

The term 'intravenous hyperalimentation' (IVH) is sometimes used, particularly outside the UK, to mean IVF. The term is rather unpopular (and inappropriate) in the UK as, clearly, one does not hyperaliment any one.

Enteral feeding

This refers to methods of supplying made-up food and nutrients through the alimentary tract by mouth, nasogastric tube, oesophagostomy, gastrostomy or duodenostomy. At present, the nutrients used for enteral feeding (p. 166) are generally manufactured and presented as a nutritional solution. This is composed of carbohydrate, fat and whole protein. However, enteral feeding may use a simpler type of nutrients in 'the elemental diet', which consists of nutrients made-up of essential parts of the food (i.e. food stuffs) such as simple carbohydrates, fatty acids, amino acids and minerals.

The principles involved in artificial feeding, be it parenteral or enteral, are similar. These two methods of feeding vary in the detail of their technique and application. Only rarely is there an absolute indication for one method of feeding to the exclusion of the other. In some cases both nutritional methods are indicated, and indeed used, in the same patient. Such cases as major excision and reconstruction of the alimentary tract are typical examples. The following report illustrates a case where both methods of artificial feeding was used.

A 56-year-old woman was admitted to the hospital with a 4-month history of dysphagia. On admission in March 1982 she could only manage to swallow thin fluids, which provoked a cough. Investigations revealed an extensive post-cricoid carcinoma of the oesophagus, involving anteriorly the larynx with almost complete obstruction of the oesophageal lumen. Her nutritional assessment showed moderately severe deficiency with negative nitrogen balance. She was fed parenterally for 8 days prior to operation, when total oesophagectomy, pharyngo-laryngectomy was carried out and the alimentary tract reconstructed using the stomach as an oesophageal substitute (pharyngo-gastric anastomosis).

A cervical gastrostomy was established at operation. Postoperatively, for 6–7 days, she was given total parenteral nutrition, followed by mixed enteral (cervical gastrostomy) feeding and IVF. By the 10th postoperative day, feeding was entirely by the enteral route using cervical gastrostomy (80% of requirement) and some oral feeding. By the 15th postoperative day, she was eating normally. On the 20th postoperative day, she was discharged.

In practice, once the need for artificial feeding is established by nutritional assessment, the method to be used is decided by taking into account the following factors:

1. The anatomical and functional integrity of the gastrointestinal tract. If there is total failure of the alimentary tract system, enteral feeding cannot be used.

2. The severity and extent of metabolic disturbances. In some cases the extent of catabolism is such that parenteral nutrition is the only method which can cope with the metabolic demands.

3. The optimum method of nutrition for a given patient in a specific situation.

4. The expertise and facilities available.
5. Cost.

A majority of patients requiring artificial nutritional support are helped by enteral methods of feeding. On the whole, enteral feeding is simpler in its application, requires less rigorous monitoring than parenteral feeding and is less costly.

However, neither the simplicity of enteral (compared with parenteral) feeding, nor its popularity (partly related to simplicity), should prevent the clinician or 'team' offering their patient the optimum treatment, if this be by parenteral feeding.

The three nutritional modalities, which can in many instances be used with clinical benefit, are normal, parenteral and enteral feeding.

8. Nutritional Assessment

A rational approach to nutritional management of a patient is correction of the existing deficiencies, and the establishment of an appropriate regime which adequately covers the requirements for the given situation. Assessment of the nutritional status of an individual enables recognition of deficiencies which can then be corrected. However, adequate nutritional assessment also allows:

- the prediction of patients most likely to require nutritional support;
- the definition of the nutritional status of a patient as a baseline for future reference;
- for the estimation of the patient's basic energy needs so that adequate nutritional support may be provided (Rich & Whitehouse, 1979).

There are a number of ways of assessing the nutritional status of an individual and these range from interview and clinical examination of the patient to complex and elaborate laboratory methods. While the recognition of starvation and advanced nutritional deficiencies may not be problematic (Fig. 2.1), the assessment of lesser nutritional deficits can be difficult. It is therefore important to consider some of the methods used in nutritional assessment, i.e. interview, clinical examination, biochemical markers and immunological indicators.

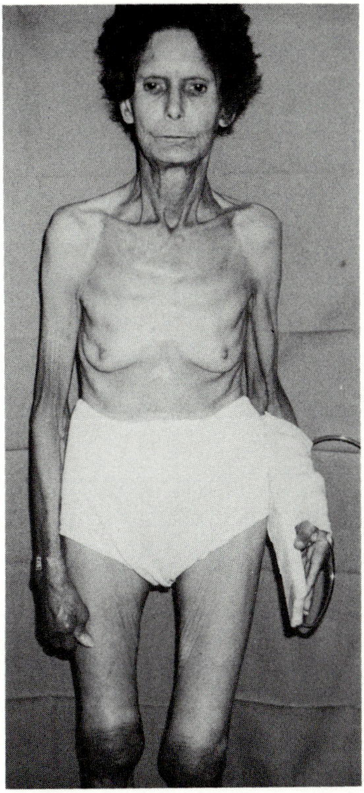

Fig. 2.1 Patient with marked malnutrition due to severe dysphagia from advanced carcinoma of the oesophagus.

INTERVIEW

The interview with the patient, and perhaps the relatives, is an important part of nutritional assessment. Malnutrition develops over a period of time and, if present, is usually the result of bizarre or inadequate eating habits. Dietary history includes details of a patient's food preferences, eating patterns, difficulties in preparing or obtaining food, and problems in eating, swallowing and retaining it. A guide to energy intake is also obtained. In 1947, Burke recommended the use of 24-hour recall of food intake, and this advice is still valid. The intake of individual nutrients may be roughly quantified by using the tables set out in the *Manual of Nutrition* (HMSO) which

Table 2.1 Clinical signs indicating nutritional status

	Normal condition	*Clinical disturbance*	*Possible disorder/deficiency*
General appearance and condition	Normal weight for height, age, sex, etc.	Overweight/underweight	Obesity/starvation
	Good muscle tone and posture	Muscle wasting/tenderness	Protein lack/Thiamin deficiency
		Haemorrhage	Vit. C deficiency
		Skeletal deformities	Vit. D deficiency
	Smooth, pink, elastic skin	Bruising/dry, rough inflamed skin	Vit. C or K/A or complex deficiency
	Normal subcutaneous tissue	Oedema	Kwashiorkor
		Fat over/under standard	Obesity/starvation
Face and head	Shiny, not easily plucked hair	Dull, dry, sparse, depigmented hair	Kwashiorkor/marasmus
	Face and neck not swollen	Moon-face/enlarged thyroid	Kwashiorkor/iodine deficiency
	Pink, healthy appearance	Nasolabial sebarrhoea	Riboflavin deficiency
	Clear, bright eyes with pink moist membranes	Dry, thickened, inflamed cornea or conjunctiva	Vit. A or B complex deficiency
		Fissures at corners	
		Corneal arcus, yellow deposits near eyes	Hyperlipidaemia
	Smooth, pink lips	Angular lesions or scars, inflammation	Riboflavin deficiency

Mouth	Red, normally rough tongue	Swollen, red, beefy tongue	Vit. B complex deficiency
		Papillary atrophy, smooth appearance	
	Healthy, red gums	Spongy, bleeding, receeding gums	Vit. C deficiency
	Bright, painfree teeth	Mottled enamel/carious teeth	Flourosis/excessive sugar
Gastrointestinal function	Good appetite and digestion	Anorexia, indigestion, diarrhoea	Niacin deficiency/may lead to deficiencies
	Normal elimination	Constipation	Inadequate fibre or fluid
	Flat abdomen	Hepato-spenomegaly	Kwashiorkor
Cardiovascular system	Normal heart rhythm/rate	Cardiac enlargement, tachycardia	Thiamin deficiency
	Normal blood pressure	Hypertension	?Sodium excess
Nervous system	Alert, responsive psychological stability	Listless, apathetic, mental confusion, depression	Vit. B complex deficiency
	Normal reflexes	Psychomotor changes	Kwashiorkor
	Normal sensory and motor nerve function	Sensory loss, paraesthesia	Thiamin deficiency
		Motor weakness, loss of some reflexes	

indicates the extent to which inadequate dietary intake can result in signs of nutritional deficiency. In addition, a well-taken dietary history will reveal specific deficiencies of nutrients which may not yet be reflected in biochemical measurements, thus enabling appropriate therapy to be given early and avoiding depletion.

CLINICAL EXAMINATION

A general physical examination provides several indicators to a patient's nutritional status. Table 2.1 indicates how various attributes may be altered through deficiency of one or more of the necessary nutrients.

Anthropometric measurements

Anthropometric measurements are useful indicators of muscle mass and body fat and, by allowing more accurate assessment, enables appropriate care to be planned for patients.

Weight/height and weight loss

Malnutrition leads to loss of weight which, when severe, is readily appreciated by patients and through simple clinical examination. Quantitation of weight loss becomes necessary when the severity of malnutrition is to be estimated. This is achieved by using standard tables of ideal weight for height and sex (Table 2.2), although these are only a guide as individuals vary considerably.

The patient is weighed in as few clothes as possible (wearing approximately the same amount of clothing on each occasion) and is measured without shoes. The actual weight is expressed as a percentage of the ideal weight (Table 2.2) which gives an indication of the severity of calorie malnutrition.

A better index of weight loss is the percentage weight change:

$$\frac{\text{Usual weight} - \text{present weight}}{\text{Usual weight}} \times 100$$

or

$$\frac{\text{Loss of weight in kg}}{\text{Usual weight in kg}} \times 100$$

A recent weight loss of 10% or more of usual weight is considered indicative of malnutrition.

Table 2.2 Desirable weights for men and women according to height and frame, based on measurements made in indoor clothing without shoes. Ages 25 years and over (*modified from Statistical Bulletin, Metropolitan Life Insurance Company (1959)*)

	Weight in kg		
Height (metres)	*Small frame*	*Medium frame*	*Large frame*
Men			
1.550	51–54	54–59	57–64
1.575	52–56	55–60	59–65
1.600	53–57	56–62	60–67
1.625	55–58	58–63	61–69
1.650	56–60	59–65	63–71
1.675	58–62	61–67	64–73
1.700	60–64	63–69	67–75
1.725	62–66	64–71	68–77
1.750	64–68	66–73	70–79
1.775	65–70	68–75	72–81
1.800	67–72	70–77	74–84
1.825	69–74	72–79	76–86
1.850	71–76	74–82	78–88
1.875	73–78	76–84	81–90
1.900	74–79	78–86	83–93
Women			
1.425	42–44	44–49	47–54
1.450	43–46	45–50	48–55
1.475	44–48	46–51	49–57
1.500	45–49	47–53	51–58
1.525	46–50	49–54	52–59
1.550	48–51	50–55	53–61
1.575	49–53	51–57	55–63
1.600	50–54	53–59	57–64
1.625	52–56	54–61	59–66
1.650	54–58	56–63	60–68
1.675	55–59	58–65	62–70
1.700	57–61	60–67	64–72
1.725	59–63	62–69	66–74
1.750	61–65	63–70	68–76
1.775	63–67	65–72	69–79

Mid-arm circumference measurement

Protein–calorie malnutrition results in muscle wastage and a reduction in subcutaneous fat deposits. The mid-arm circumference measurement, and its comparison with normal standards (Table 2.3),

Table 2.3 Adult anthropometric standards (Jelliffe, 1966)

	Sex	*Standard*	90% *Standard*	80% *Standard*	70% *Standard*	60% *Standard*
Mid-arm circumference—adults (cm)	Male	29.3	26.3	23.4	20.5	17.6
	Female	28.5	25.7	22.8	20.0	17.1
Triceps skin-fold thickness—adults (mm)	Male	12.5	11.3	10.0	8.8	7.5
	Female	16.5	14.9	13.2	11.6	9.9
Mid-arm circumference—adults (cm)	Male	25.3	22.8	20.2	17.7	15.2
	Female	23.2	20.9	18.6	16.2	13.9

indicates the degree of wastage. This measurement is carried out using a tape measure around the upper arm at the mid-point between the acromial process of the scapula and the olecranon process of the ulna (Figs 2.2a,b). To obtain accurate results, the technique is as follows:

1. If possible, measurements should be carried out by the same person.
2. The patient's nondominant (usually left) arm is used and the forearm flexed at a 90° angle.
3. The mid-point of the arm is marked and regular measurements made posteriorly at the same point (Fig. 2.2c).
4. A nonstretchable tape measure is used and positioned snugly (not pulled tight) around the arm (Fig. 2.2d).
5. The reading is recorded in centimetres and millimetres.

The measurements are compared firstly with normal standards (Table 2.3) and then with the patient's previous records.

Skin-fold thickness

This is a simple estimate of subcutaneous fat which reduces, and may eventually disappear, in malnutrition. It can be measured at several sites (the triceps, biceps, sub-scapula or supra-iliac sites), but the triceps skin-fold thickness (TSF) is most commonly used. A skin-fold caliper is used for the measurement which is carried out at the point already marked on the posterior side of the upper arm (Figs 2.3a,b). This measurement requires some practice to obtain proficiency, although once the skill is acquired it is a quick and easy technique to undertake. It is therefore desirable to take two or three measurements and record the average. The measurement is compared with normal standards (Table 2.3).

Mid-arm muscle circumference

This measurement gives a good indication of the lean body mass and, therefore, of skeletal protein reserves. It is calculated from two previous measurements by the following formula:

$$\text{Arm muscle circumference (cm)} = \text{Arm circumference (cm)} - (0.314 \times \text{triceps skinfold (mm)})$$

The anthropometric measurements are, if possible, carried out by

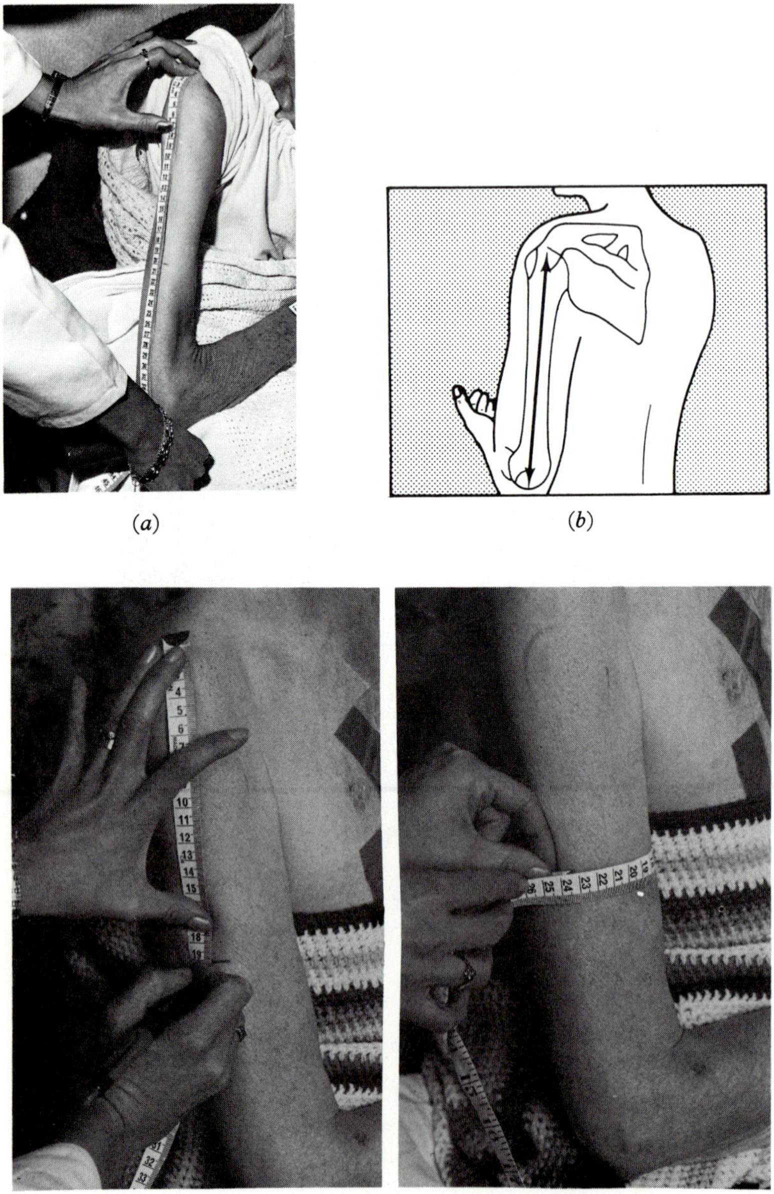

Fig. 2.2 Measuring the mid-arm circumference. (a), (b) Determining the mid-point of the arm. (c) Marking the point for taking the measurement. (d) Measuring the circumference.

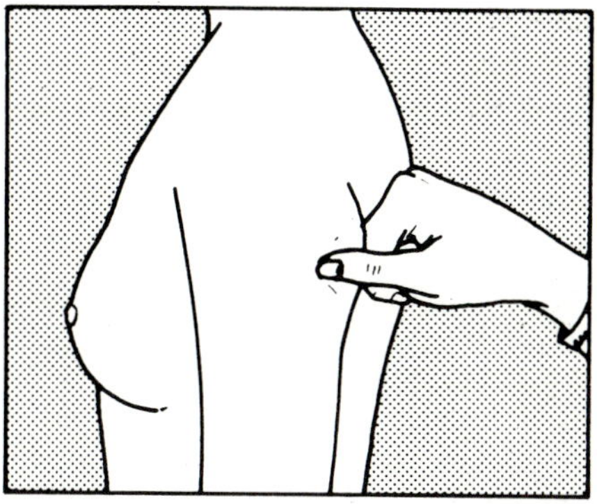

(*a*)

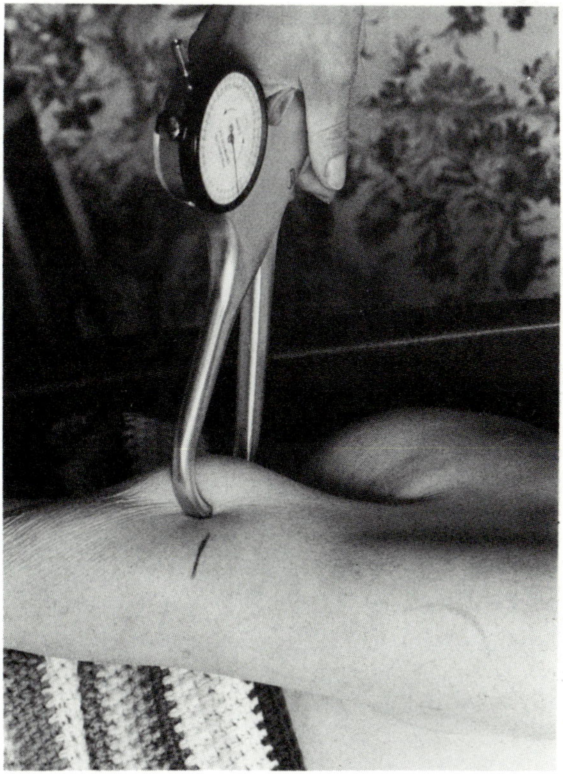

(*b*)

Fig. 2.3 (*a*) *Taking up a fold of skin to apply caliper.* (*b*) *Measuring triceps skinfold thickness, using a skin caliper.*

the same person as there may be considerable variation between measurements performed by different people. Table 2.3 shows the adult standards for the three anthropometric measurements usually carried out on patients. It is usually accepted that a measure of below 90% of standard indicates moderate malnutrition, while severe malnutrition is present if it is below 60%. However, these standards have not been developed from a British population and there is some debate about their value.

However, all the anthropometric measurements discussed here are non-invasive and relatively simple to use, once practised and competence achieved, and are of value in many situations. These measurements, compared to standards, help identify the status of different body tissues, changes in which may not otherwise be recognized. The following data obtained from 3 patients (Coates, 1983) illustrate this point.

Patient 1. In this patient, obesity masked a degree of protein depletion.

Weight	121.0% of ideal weight
Triceps skin-fold thickness	268.0% of standard
Upper arm circumference	114.0% of standard
Arm muscle circumference	90.0% of standard

Patient 2 was overweight, and a reducing diet has been prescribed, although other measurements indictated a moderate degree of protein loss and a severe degree of depletion of fat stores. The excess weight was due to retained fluid.

Weight	116.0% of ideal weight
Triceps skin-fold thickness	27.0% of standard
Upper arm circumference	70.0% of standard
Arm muscle circumference	80.0% of standard

Patient 3 was suffering from a chronic, rather than an acute, illness and had fat stores that were depleted to a greater extent than the muscle mass. This is a physiologically valuable adaptation to reduced food intake over a long period of time.

Weight	72.0% of ideal weight
Triceps skin fold	27.0% of standard
Upper arm circumference	65.0% of standard
Arm muscle circumference	74.0% of standard

BIOCHEMICAL MARKERS

There are a variety of biochemical tests which reveal certain aspects of nutritional deficiencies. Some of the more commonly used are set out below.

Total plasma proteins

These are reduced only in severe degrees of deficiency.

Plasma albumin

By virtue of the colloid osmotic pressure they exert, albumins are important constituents of plasma. Their reduction introduces an imbalance between the intravascular and extravascular interstitial fluid compartments of the body, resulting in the expansion of the latter with resulting oedema in severe cases. The albumins are reduced in nutritional deficiency.

Other plasma proteins, such as transferrin (proteins involved in iron binding) and pre-albumins, are altered earlier in protein malnutrition.

Other biochemical markers

Urinary excretion of 3-methyl histidine is a measure of the muscle protein participating in metabolic turnover, creatinine/height index and changes in the plasma amino acid profile are also indicators of protein status.

Nitrogen balance studies

Reference has been made to nitrogen balance studies designed to calculate the nitrogen intake and output (p. 37). Output, in the absence of abnormal losses (diarrhoea and fistula), is measured by determining the nitrogen content of the urinary output over a period of 24 hours.

Collection and measurement of 24-hour output is effected and accurately recorded. On the day of study, the bladder is emptied (say at 9 a.m.) and the urine omitted. Thereafter, the patient is asked to pass urine into a container. The volume is measured and recorded, and put into a container with a preservative provided by the laboratory. At 9 a.m. the following day the bladder is emptied and the urine included in the 24-hour collection.

Nitrogen loss in urine is calculated as follows:

$$\text{N loss in urine} = \text{24 hr urine urea (g)} \times \frac{28}{60} \times \frac{6}{5}$$

The factor of $\frac{28}{60}$ is allowing for the fact that the gram molecular weight of urea is 60 and it contains 28 g of nitrogen. The fraction of $\frac{6}{5}$ corrects for the $\frac{1}{5}$ of nitrogen losses through the kidneys as substances other than urea.

A more accurate assessment of nitrogen loss (Lee, 1974) can be obtained by making a number of corrections in the figure obtained from the above formula. A correction for changes in blood urea can be made as follows:

$$\text{Change in blood urea (mmol/l)} \times 0.028 \times 60\% \text{ body weight (estimate of total body water)}$$

A further allowance will be made for protein loss in urine or other body fluids. The amount of protein lost divided by 6.25 will give the nitrogen lost in these fluids. In addition, 1 to 1.5 g of nitrogen is lost in faeces and skin.

Thus, an estimate of total nitrogen loss is obtained by adding:

nitrogen loss in urine
\+ correction for rise in blood urea (subtracted if blood urea falls)
\+ Nitrogen lost as protein in body fluids
\+ Allowance for losses in skin and faeces

Nitrogen intake is measured by weighing the protein included in a patient's diet over a 24-hour period, subtracting from it that not eaten and calculating the nitrogen content (6.25 g of protein contains 1 g of nitrogen). Nitrogen balance is calculated by subtracting the nitrogen lost from the body from the amount ingested.

The body is said to be in nitrogen equilibrium when the nitrogen intake and output are equal in amount. It is said to be in negative nitrogen balance when the output is greater than the intake. Nitrogen balance is positive when the intake is superior to the output, indicating that protein is being laid down within the body.

A negative nitrogen balance signifies that some of the body's proteins, primarily those of muscular tissues, are broken down and metabolized as a source of energy and the nitrogen residue excreted in the urine. Nitrogen excretion in excess of intake is thus an index of the body's protein breakdown, principally the muscles, as it is used for energy in general body metabolism.

IMMUNOLOGICAL MARKERS

In order to appreciate the significance of immunological tests in nutritional assessment, some of the principles of the immune response are outlined below.

Historically, immunity is defined as resistance to infection. In its more general sense, immunity or the immune response is when the body recognizes a foreign protein material (an antigen) and responds to it by producing antibodies, which tend to eliminate or neutralize the antigen effect, or react to it in some specific way. The manifestations of the antigen and antibody encounters are complicated and varied. Protection against infection after vaccination, graft rejection and hypersensitivity reactions are all manifestations of the immune response and are due to the formation of the antigen–antibody complex. Tissues involved in the immune response include white blood cells, lymphoid tissues, the thymus gland and the reticulo-endothelial system.

Among many factors influencing the immune response of the body is the nutritional state. It is therefore not surprising that immunological testing is designed to assess nutritional deficiencies.

Skin testing

These tests are based on the delayed-type hypersensitivity reaction in which an intradermal injection of an antigen causes localized oedema and inflammation in a responsive (previously sensitized) subject. The principle on which these tests are based is that the majority of the population react to certain antigens to which they have been previously exposed, but that in certain circumstances (e.g. cancer cachexia and malnutrition) they fail to do so. This state of unresponsiveness, or anergy, appears to be associated with severe malnutrition. The three antigens commonly used in the UK in connection with nutritional assessment are tuberculin, candida albicans and streptokinase antigen. Some investigations use five or more antigens at the same time. The total lack of response is referred to as anergy.

Immunoglobulins

Immunoglobulins are proteins and are important components in the immunological competence of the body. They are in fact the so-called circulatory antibodies. However, they are relatively unimportant as markers for nutritional deficiencies.

Lymphocytes

The lymphocytes are important in antibody production. The total lymphocyte count therefore becomes part of nutritional assessment.

PRACTICAL ASSESSMENT

All patients need their nutritional status assessed. For many, the complete battery of tests described above is completely unnecessary and expensive. However, those who are candidates for enteral or parenteral feeding do require a great number of tests, but the full range is likely to be used only in research.

Some of the common markers of malnutrition are listed in Table 2.4.

Table 2.4 Common indices of calorie/protein malnutrition

Ideal weight	Less than 60%
Weight loss (% weight changes)	Greater than 10%
Triceps skin-fold	Less than 10 mm in males Less than 13 mm in females
Mid-arm circumference	Less than 23.0 cm in males Less than 22.0 cm in females
Serum albumin	Less than 35 g/l
Serum protein	Less than 60 g/l
Serum transferrin	Less than 1.5 g/l
Cell mediated immunity (skin test to antigens)	Candida skin tests negative and tuberculin skin tests negative
Lymphocyte count	Less than $1500/10^{-6}$ l
Nitrogen balance	Negative

Anthropometric measurements, clinical examination and interview are all readily carried out by anyone involved in nutritional assessment, with a proviso on the competence of the assessor (p. 59), and are usually adequate for many patients. Some of the plasma proteins (e.g. transferrin) are readily measured by a laboratory and used when a more detailed assessment is needed. Nitrogen balance studies are not difficult in principle, but accurately estimating the nitrogen intake and ensuring that all urine is collected for the 24-hour period may cause difficulties that reduce its value as a routine measurement.

9. Nursing Patients Receiving Artificial Feeding

Nurses play an important role in the specific management of enteral or parenteral feeding, and this is discussed where appropriate. However, the nursing involvement is considerably greater than this.

ASSESSMENT

A nurse's involvement with patients and relatives begins with a patient's admission to hospital, when she carries out the nursing assessment to identify problems and potential problems (McFarlane and Castledine, 1982). In taking the patient's nursing history, the nurse needs to find out about the patient's normal life-style and the way activities of daily living have been dealt with, and the alterations that have occurred as a result of illness. It is particularly important to find out about nutrient and fluid intake in these patients, together with any physical, psychological and social factors that may influence nutrition. Information about normal bowel function is also needed. Assessment is also made of patients' knowledge and understanding of their condition. In addition, nurses also carry out an assessment of the patient's physical condition, with particular reference to those aspects relevant to nursing. Condition of skin and hair, presence of oedema, signs of weight loss or dehydration, condition of mouth and breathlessness all indicate nutritional or fluid disturbances, and are easily assessed whilst giving nursing care. On admission, all patients are weighed and their height measured to allow an assessment of their ideal weight; any marked deviation is noted and recorded. Some nurses should also become able to carry out anthropometric measurements to assess a patient's nutritional status more precisely.

IDENTIFICATION OF PROBLEMS

With knowledge about the patient (obtained from the assessment), the disorder and the expected treatment, nurses identify problems and plan appropriate nursing care. These problems are considered in three groups:

1. Patients' problems associated with the need for artificial nutrition.
2. Patients' problems associated with receiving artificial nutrition.
3. Potential problems associated with artificial feeding.

Patients' problems associated with need for artificial nutrition

People admitted to hospital are likely to be anxious about the new and strange environment in the hospital, the ward routine, 'what is and will be happening to them', and their possible diagnosis and prognosis. In addition, loss of control over events happening to them add to their anxiety. Those requiring artificial feeding are likely to be particularly anxious, especially if they have lost a considerable amount of weight in a short time, which many people associate with severe illness. Psychological care to minimize anxiety is an important part of nursing, requiring sensitivity to the patient's verbal and non-verbal cues. The ability to listen, understand and demonstrate this understanding is essential. Clearly, nurses are the best people to give information and teach patients about various activities and procedures related to their care.

Patients who are malnourished and possibly dehydrated, with the skin in poor condition, may also be oedematous due to the fall in plasma proteins which accompanies severe malnutrition. All these factors increase the risk of developing pressure sores. The risk is even greater if mobility is reduced due to weakness, or if the artificial feeding itself 'ties' them to their beds. Regular changing of position is necessary to relieve prolonged pressure on one area. The most effective way of achieving this is to teach patients the importance of frequently shifting their position. If this is not possible, then a patient will require at least 2-hourly turning. The use of sheepskins and other aids is also of value to distribute weight over a larger area. While cleanliness is important, the skin may be dry and scaly, due to a deficiency in essential fatty acids or vitamins, and soap is therefore used in moderation. The application of a moisturizing cream or oil improves the condition of heels, elbows and sacral area, and helps make a patient more confortable. Spirit is a drying agent and is not used on pressure areas. It is very important to prevent any development of pressure sores as the healing of a wound is likely to be retarded in malnourished patients.

Patients may feel weak and become quickly exhausted when active and their care therefore needs to be organized to give adequate periods of rest. A short rest after the bed bath, for instance, may help a patient to face with equanimity the prospect of getting out of bed and walking a short distance.

In patients unable to eat normally, particularly in the presence of dehydration, bowel function may be disturbed. Although a large part of the faecal bulk is made up of cell debris and bacteria, etc., lack of food and fluid intake is likely to result in constipation. Many patients are distressed by this and it can be managed with suppositories to establish regular bowel function.

Mouth care is also important, particularly if oral fluids are not taken, although patients receiving enteral and parenteral feeding are likely to have a moist, clean mouth once dehydration has been corrected (Howarth, 1977).

In malnutrition, an individual's immune response is compromised. The patient is at risk of developing infection and therefore care is always taken to minimize exposure to pathogenic organisms. Ensuring a patient has a daily bath and clean linen at frequent intervals, as well as washing one's hands thoroughly between caring for different patients, all help to minimize the risk of transmitting infective organisms. Malnourished patients should not be placed in a bed next to others with overt infections, and any other factors known to reduce the immune response are minimized (e.g. stress, resulting from anxiety, which influences the immune response by the effect of corticosteroid hormones). Anxiety is minimized by giving information to help a patient understand his surroundings and the events which are taking place. Developing a relationship with the patient will encourage him to ask questions and talk about his anxieties, which will help him to relax and fit into the strange environment of the ward.

Problems associated with receiving artificial feeding

Many of these problems tend to be specific to the method of feeding in use, and are discussed where appropriate.

Once a parenteral feeding system is set up, it causes no discomfort (if all goes well), though a patient receiving enteral feeding may find the nasogastric tube uncomfortable in the nose and at the back of the throat. The nasogastric tube needs to be firmly positioned, but fixing it along the nose and the forehead may be uncomfortable and make the wearing of spectacles impossible. Attaching the tube to the nose and cheek is probably preferable for most patients (p. 173). The fine bore tubes now available for enteral feeding cause much less discomfort but, because these patients may be unable to take oral fluid and foods, frequent mouthwashes are needed to keep mouths fresh. Even with patients allowed nothing by mouth, rubbing a slice of lemon on the lips and tongue will prevent drying of the mouth.

Gastrointestinal disturbances may arise in those receiving enteral feeding. Nausea, abdominal distension, diarrhoea or constipation may develop and are further discussed on p. 185. Patients with diarrhoea require sympathetic care, with ready access to a toilet or commode. If soreness develops around the anus, a barrier cream is applied.

Patients receiving parenteral nutrition, and those having enteral feeding on a continuous feed system, will find their mobility restricted by the equipment. Patients who are fit, however, are often able to walk around pushing a wheeled intravenous stand, carrying their feed with them (Fig. 2.4). When strong enough, patients are able to wash themselves, etc., and, with supervision, are able to have a bath. Care is needed to keep the site of insertion of the central venous line dry.

A particularly important group of problems are psychological ones associated with an inability to eat normally and a change in body image. Eating a meal is usually a social occasion involving interaction with others. Deprivation of this, and the reminder at every meal-time that one is not eating normally, may result in despondency. Arranging activities so that the patient is in another part of the ward at mealtimes or, if possible, arranging for relatives or friends to visit at mealtimes to distract the patient, is helpful.

Some patients have difficulty in adjusting to the change in body

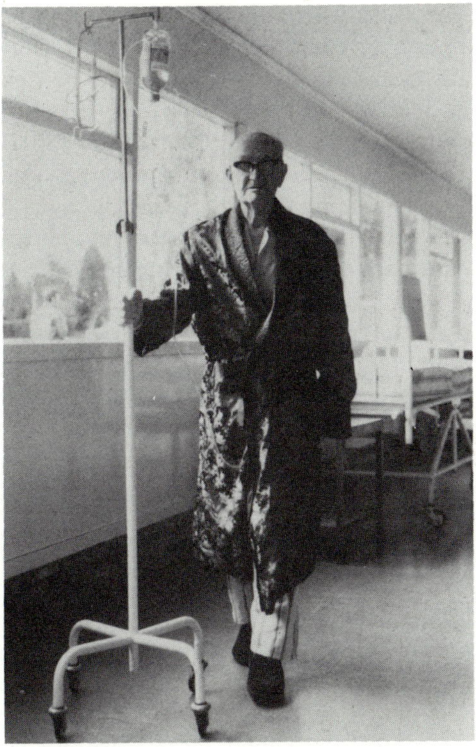

Fig. 2.4 An ambulent patient with intravenous feeding in progress.

image associated with the presence of tubes and the loss of ability to feed normally. These patients need encouragement and support; helping female patients to wash and set their hair and apply make up, for instance, or getting male patients to shave everyday, will help to improve morale. These aspects of care are more effectively given when a patient assignment system of ward organization is used, allowing the patient to get to know his nurse over a period of time. On the other hand, those who have been unable to eat normally for some time may be so relieved to be receiving nourishment that these changes are usually accepted with equanimity.

Potential Problems Associated with Artificial Feeding

These problems are mainly discussed (with specific details of management) in chapters 16, 22. The nurse's role in this area is concerned with recognizing problems at an early stage and organizing care to abort any complications.

Therefore, to identify problems at an early stage, careful observation and accurate recording is essential. To aid recognition of infection these patients have their temperature, pulse and respiration recorded regularly, ensuring that the thermometer is left in position for the 7 minutes needed to accurately measure oral temperature, or 10 minutes in the axilla (Nichols and Kucha, 1972; Nichols *et al.*, 1966). Some of these patients need 4-hourly observations, including blood pressure measurement, for others, twice daily TPR recordings are adequate. Body temperature is best measured between 7–8 p.m., followed by 5–6 p.m., as a rise in temperature is most likely to be observed during these hours. Temperature measurement is less sensitive between 7–8 a.m. and 3–4 p.m. and routine measurement should therefore be avoided during these times of day (Angerami, 1980).

An accurate measurement and recording of fluid intake and output, and regular urine testing, is also very important to ensure correct intake and help identify fluid and electrolyte disturbances. Unfortunately, there is considerable variation in the way fluid balance charts are completed, and the care with which they are done. Because of these variations, particularly in the way intravenous intake is recorded, it is necessary to be absolutely clear about the practice on a particular ward. Considerable inaccuracies will arise over a 24-hour period if intake and output are not measured accurately.

Another potential problem may arise when artificial feeding is being discontinued. It is not uncommon to find appetite is poor, and food intake low, when artificial feeding is first discontinued. It is during this period that a patient may again go into negative nitrogen balance and his condition deteriorates. Therefore, encouragement to eat, and reassurance that appetite will return, are needed. Also careful observation and recording of food actually eaten is important. When food is inadequate for a patient's needs, then nutritional supplements are given.

ORGANIZATION OF CARE OF PATIENTS RECEIVING ARTIFICIAL FEEDING

The management of patients receiving artificial nutrition can be organized in several different ways, but the care required falls into two main areas: (1) the specific management of the artificial feeding system and administration of nutrients, and (2) the general nursing care of the patient.

Specific management of the artificial feeding system is also arranged in different ways. In some hospitals, particularly in North America, a fairly large nutritional team deals entirely with the artificial feeding, even taking responsibility for changing the bottles of nutrient solution. Elsewhere, a nutritional team, including a specialist nurse, undertakes assessment, gives advice on the nutritional management of a patient and undertakes the necessary teaching of staff, sometimes taking additional responsibility for patients with considerable and complex nutritional disturbances. Expert advice may also be available on a much less formal basis when individual members of staff, medical and nursing, become interested and develop their expertise in this area. Colleagues may then ask for advice as required. An extension of this is found where a specialist nurse nutritionist, or a nurse with a special responsibility for teaching new staff, becomes highly knowledgeable and skilled and acts as a resource person for ward staff. Finally, a ward sister may find herself with a patient requiring artificial feeding and no one available with the specific nursing expertise needed to help her. While nutritional programmes and technical aspects can be dealt with by medical staff, the ward sister only has published work to refer to as regards the nursing management required.

In the UK, the hospital nutritional team rarely takes over complete responsibility for artificial feeding. Therefore, on every ward where such feeding is in progress, a ward sister and other trained staff are responsible for ensuring a patient safely receives the correct care. How is this achieved? Clearly, the first requisite is that trained staff have the adequate knowledge needed, and every qualified nurse should consider herself professionally responsible for keeping that knowledge up-to-date.

Nursing work on wards in the UK is organized in a number of different ways, although Pembrey (1980) found that in many wards there was no recognizable system of management. The aim is, of course, to give the patient the care he requires. Some aspects of care (e.g. psychological support) are most easily given when one nurse has the responsibility for the majority of general care. Therefore, she and the patient get to know each other. The patient also requires the technical care associated with artificial feeding, some of which carries risks with definite morbidity, even mortality (p. 151). These techniques are complex and must be carried out by someone with the necessary expertise. To achieve both of these ends, some formal management is required and the ward sister has to consider the advantages and disadvantages of different organizational styles. Patient and task assignment, team nursing and primary nursing are the alternative methods currently under discussion in the study of ward management.

Pembrey (1980) found that 82% of ward sisters did not organize the work according to a patient's individual needs and the skills of different members of staff. Clearly, if patients having artificial feeding are to receive the correct care, then both of these factors must be considered when allocating work.

Patient assignment

In the UK, more wards are moving towards a patient assignment system of organization. Ideally each nurse is allocated to the same patients for a period of time to allow the development of a nurse–patient relationship. She gives the nursing care, under the general supervision of the ward sister, and is in an ideal position to give the psychological support required, even though she may also need some support herself. However, where the ward has a number of patients receiving artificial feeding, and has the usual mixture of senior and junior nurses in training and some (but probably not enough) trained staff, this system is difficult to administer. There may not be enough senior staff, who have quite specifically been taught the techniques involved, to give the total nursing care for all the patients on artificial feeding.

Task assignment

In using a task assignment system of organization, each nurse is allocated to carry out particular tasks for a large number of patients. This makes it very difficult for a patient to get to know any one nurse well, and so receive the psychological care required. It is also easy for some patient needs to be missed if the ward sister has omitted to allocate some one to carry out the necessary care. Using this system, there is little scope for nurses in training to think and learn about the care of the whole patient. In addition, there is the possible disadvantage of increasing the risk of transmitting infection from patient to patient. However, it does allow the allocation of trained, or at least senior student nurses taught and supervised in practice, to carry out the skilled technical care required in the management of artificial feeding.

Team nursing

Neither patient nor task assignment appear entirely satisfactory and therefore a combination of the two within a team nursing system of organization may be more advantageous. The allocation of a senior nurse, as team leader, and junior nurses to care for a group of patients can work well. The junior nurses are allocated to individual patients within the group, and give the general care. The senior nurse supervises, teaches and helps them as needed, and carries out the technical care required with the assistance of the junior nurse allocated to that patient. In this system, both the general (including psychological) and technical nursing needs of a patient receiving artificial feeding can be satisfied.

Primary nursing

In this system of nursing organization, a registered nurse is allocated a number of patients for whom she is responsible during their stay in hospital. She assesses, plans and evaluates their care and, when on duty, is involved in the implementation of this plan. Other nurses assist her by carrying out her plan when she is off-duty. Nurses in training work under the supervision of a primary nurse in all aspects of the nursing process. This system probably affords the best opportunity for giving high quality patient care (MacFarlane and Castledine, 1982).

Whichever system of organization is used, the nurse is accountable to either the team leader or ward sister for the care she gives. The team leaders report directly to the ward sister about the condition of patients and the care given to those for whom she is responsible. The ward sister has to be certain that patients are not at risk because the staff are unsure about procedures to be carried out. On wards where artificial feeding is in progress, it is useful to have a copy of the agreed procedures involved in the care of these patients. Newly allocated staff must have specific teaching about the care required.

REFERENCES

Angerami E. (1980). Epidemiological study of body temperature in patients in a teaching hospital. *Int. J. Nurs. Stud.*; **17**: 91–99.

Burke B.S. (1947). The dietary history as a tool in research. *Journal of American Dietetic Association*; **23**: 1041–1046.

Coates V. (1983). Unpublished M.Phil. Thesis. Univ. of Hull.

Cuthbertson D.P. (1980). Historical background to parenteral nutrition. Symposia, 1st European Congress on Parenteral and Enteral Nutrition (1979) (Wahren J. ed.) *Acta Chirurgica Scand. Supplement*; **498**.

Howarth H. (1977). Mouth care procedures for the very ill. *Nursing Times*; **73**: 354–355.

Lee H.A. (1974). *Parenteral Nutrition in Acute Metabolic Illness.* London, New York: Academic Press.

McFarlane of Llandaff, Castledine G. (1982). *A Guide to the Practice of Nursing Using the Nursing Progress.* London: C.V. Mosby Co.

Nichols G.A., Kucha D.H. (1972). Taking adult temperatures: oral measurements. *Am. J. Nurs.*; **72**: 1091–1093.

Nichols G.A., Ruskin M.M., Glor B.A.K., Kelly W.H. (1966). Oral, axillary and rectal temperature determinations and relationships. *Nursing Research*; **15**: 307–310.

Pembrey S. (1980). *The Ward Sister: Key to Nursing.* London: Royal College of Nursing.

Rich A.J., Whitehouse M.E. (1979). The relevance of pre-operative nutritional assessment. In *Developments in Clinical Nutrition* (Johnston I.D.A., Lee H.A. eds.) Proceedings of a Symposium held in London, Oct. 1978.

FURTHER READING

Ballinger W.F., Collins J.A., Drucker W.R., Dudrick S.J., Zeppa R. (1975). *Manual of Surgical Nutrition.* Philadelphia: W.B. Saunders.

Bennion M. (1979). *Clinical Nutrition.* New York: Harper and Row.

Bistrian B.R., Blackburn G.L., Hallowell E., Heddle R. (1974). Protein status of general surgical patients. *JAMA*; **230**(6): 858–860.

Blackburn G.L., Bistrian B.R., Maini B.S., Schlamm H.T., Smith M.F. (1977). Nutritional and metabolic assessment of the hospitalized patient. *J. Parent. and Ent. Nutr.*; **1**: 11–22.

Blackburn G.L., Thornton P.A. (1979). Nutritional assessment of the hospitalized patient. *Med. Clin. of N. Am.*; **63**(5): 1103–1115.

Fischer J.E. (1980). Nutritional support in the seriously ill patient. *Cur. Prob. Surg.*; **17**(19): 466–532.

Goode A.W. (1981). The scientific basis of nutritional assessment. *Br. J. Anaesth.*; **53**(2): 161–167.

Hill G., Blacket R., Pickford I., Birkinshaw L., Young G., Warren J., Schorah C., Morgan D. (1977). Malnutrition in surgical patients. *Lancet*; **1**: 689–692.

Michigan Nurses Association—Curn Project (1981). *Using Research to Improve Nursing Practice: Distress Reduction Through Sensory Preparation.* New York: Grune and Stratton.

Wolfe B.M., Phillips G.J., Hodges R.E. (1979). Evaluation and management of nutritional status before surgery. *Med. Clin. of N. Am.*; **63**(6): 1257–1269.

Yarborough M.F., Curreri M.D. (1981). *Surgical Nutrition.* Edinburgh: Churchill Livingstone.

SECTION III

Parenteral Nutrition

This section considers the supply of nutrients to patients via the intravenous route. The clinical development of parenteral nutrition occurred earlier than enteral feeding (Section IV), but both discussions follow the same plan.

The selection of patients and indications for use are discussed first, followed by a consideration of nutrient solutions available. Methods of delivery and the equipment required are discussed in detail, and monitoring of therapy is considered. Finally, complications associated with parenteral feeding, and their prevention, are outlined. Throughout, nursing implications are emphasized. Some detail may be seen as more appropriate to medical than to nursing staff, but this is intentional because of the central role the nurse plays not only in the care of the patient, but also in the ordering of equipment and management of the regime.

10. Introduction

The term 'parenteral nutrition' is applied to methods which provide food stuffs and other essential requirements of the body by a route other than that of the alimentary tract. For practical purposes this has become synonymous with intravenous feeding although, in its wider application, it also includes the sometimes used subcutaneous route.

Clinical intravenous feeding has been in use for less than 50 years, but the idea of intravenous infusion goes back to the 17th century. Documentation is not precise as to who first attempted, or successfully managed, to infuse fluid into man's circulation, but historical reviews leave little doubt that blood transfusions had been attempted long before the infusion of fluid or nutrients.

The first recorded intravenous infusion is attributed to Sir Christopher Wren who, in the 1650s, injected wine, beer and drugs into a dog's vein. Shortly after, in the 1660s, Richard Lower of Oxford and Jean Baptiste Denis of Montpelier (physician to King Louis the 14th of France) carried out a blood transfusion from animal to man. This primitive and yet significant experiment paved the way, but was not applied to the clinical practice of intravenous infusion. The latter had to wait for the development of more sophisticated techniques, and advances in other directions and disciplines. Most significant and relevant was the discovery of the microbial origin of infection by Louis Pasteur, and the development of asepsis by Sir Joseph Lister.

Early in the 20th century, several workers successfully infused solutions of saline, dextrose and protein hydrolysate. Understanding of the metabolic response to trauma, resulting from the work of Sir David Cuthbertson (1930), and its application to surgery, notably by Moore (1959), have been a great stimulus in intravenous feeding. The last 25 years have seen the emergence and expansion of indications for parenteral nutrition in medicine and surgery. More advanced and safe techniques of infusion have now been designed to reduce the incidence of complications. Better understanding of animal and human physiology, together with metabolic requirements in specific circumstances, have also allowed a more precise application of intravenous feeding. In addition, a major advance has been made in the manufacture of nutrient solutions. Consequently, the intravenous route has become a well established and accepted method of feeding. However, for all its widespread acceptance, parenteral nutrition is not to be regarded as a simple method of intravenous infusion to be applied without careful planning and/or definite indications. It is a therapeutic measure requiring knowledge and understanding in its application and aims. In practice, this involves:

- Selection of patients for intravenous feeding.
- Assessment of nutritional requirements and selection of nutrient solution to satisfy the patient's needs.
- Delivery of nutrient solutions to patients, including the technical aspects.
- Care of infusion system.
- Monitoring parenteral nutrition therapy.
- Knowledge of complications and their prevention.

Clearly, parenteral nutrition is not successfully undertaken without careful planning and coordinated team work. The nursing staff in their everyday duties are involved in all stages of intravenous feeding.

11. Selection of Patients for Intravenous Feeding

Parenteral nutrition is indicated in a variety of medical and surgical cases in which a patient's nutritional requirements cannot be met through the alimentary tract. The patients requiring such nutrition are often very ill and require skilled nursing care, one element of which is nutritional management. The patient's need for parenteral nutrition is usually due to difficulty in ingestion of food or inability to absorb food stuffs. Alternatively, the body's requirements might be increased to such an extent that the alimentary tract cannot keep pace with the high metabolic turnover.

Patients with obstructive lesions of the oesophagus, total dysphagia and severe nutritional difficulties, are obvious candidates for intravenous nutrition, as are those with frequent vomiting due to pyloric stenosis.

Following extensive trauma and surgery, the circulatory system is normally the only suitable route for the delivery and assimilation of nutrients. Therefore, this group of patients may also require intravenous feeding. In addition, this method of feeding is important in helping to get patients into a fit state to cope with the metabolic demands of major surgery. With the principles outlined above, intravenous feeding is used for the following reasons:

1. After major and extensive surgery.
2. In pre-operative preparation of patients undergoing surgery for alimentary tract malignancies.
3. In burns and extensive injuries.
4. In cases of alimentary tract disorders and failure.
5. In severe infections.
6. In hypercatabolic states when nutritional needs are greatly increased.
7. Where there is need for nutritional support, an example of which is as an adjunct to cancer chemotherapy.

In practice, patients are selected for parenteral nutrition after due consideration is given to:

- The type of condition from which they are suffering.
- When normal feeding is either impossible or definitely inadequate.
- When the choice of artificial nutrition has been made, and it has been decided that enteral feeding is either impractical or otherwise less beneficial to the patient.

PARENTERAL NUTRITION AFTER EXTENSIVE SURGERY

Any trauma, including a surgical operation, introduces a temporary metabolic disturbance (p. 38). The extent and duration of the metabolic disturbance depends on the severity of surgical trauma and the presence of any complications.

Parenteral nutrition is thus an important therapeutic tool in operations on the gastrointestinal tract, or when any postoperative surgical complications involve the digestive system. These include paralytic ileus, peritonitis and anastomotic leak, in which intravenous feeding has a life-saving role as, in many of these conditions, the alimentary tract is unusable.

In these instances, the postoperative catabolic phase is minimized, or checked, by providing the patient with an extra nutritional allowance, which is best supplied by the intravenous route. When a surgical operation involves the alimentary tract itself, the post-operative parenteral supply of nutrients becomes mandatory, at least for a few days.

Minor surgical operations entail minimal and very temporary metabolic aberrations which, in the absence of complications, necessitate no parenteral or additional artificial nutrition. Following surgery, normal feeding is resumed within a few days with no ill effects as long as sufficient volume of fluid is provided. Even in many of the major surgical procedures, such as operations on the lungs (e.g. pneumonectomy), there is no place for intravenous alimentation in spite of high postoperative metabolic demands. This is due to the fact that there are usually no pre-operative deficiencies found in these patients and, almost immediately after operation, normal oral feeding is resumed. However, when a major operative procedure is envisaged in patients who have considerable nutritional deficiences, intravenous feeding is necessary.

PARENTERAL NUTRITION IN PRE-OPERATIVE PREPARATION

For some time now it has become clear that the nutritional preparation of patients plays an important part in both their operability and their chance of uncomplicated recovery.

In practice, it is necessary to evaluate the nutritional state of a patient, and correct the deficiencies, before judging suitability for a proposed operation. This generalization, however, applies particularly to those who, by the very nature of their condition, become undernourished and who require surgical intervention. Nowhere is this more obvious than in a patient suffering from a malignant upper alimentary tract obstruction, such as carcinoma of the oesophagus.

The following case illustrates this point.

In 1976 a 68-year-old man was admitted to hospital on account of severe dysphagia. He could not swallow his saliva without difficulty and was in severe nutritional deficiency (Fig. 3.1a), with loss of weight, low serum protein and albumin, low haemoglobin and high blood urea. He was in negative nitrogen balance. His barium swallow x-rays showed almost complete obstruction of the oesophagus (Fig. 3.1b), and the endoscopic examination confirmed the presence of lower oesophageal and upper gastric cancer. He was given total parenteral feeding for 12 days, with high calorie and nitrogen content. He was also given two units of blood. (The effectiveness of this treatment is shown in Fig. 3.1c.) He was then submitted to operation. This entailed partial oesophagectomy, total gastrectomy, splenectomy (Fig. 3.1d) and reconstruction of the alimentary tract by oesophagojejunal and jejunojejunal anastomosis (Roux-en-y). His recovery was uneventful and he was discharged home 18 days after his operation. Figure 3.1e,f show him and his barium swallow examination 5 years after operation.

PARENTERAL NUTRITION IN BURNS

Several factors are responsible for patients with severe burns generally qualifying for artificial nutrition and, more specifically, for parenteral nutrition. Firstly, extensive burns involve much tissue destruction resulting in high metabolic demands. Secondly, and more essentially, the protective skin is damaged and there is an outpouring of protein-rich fluid. Additionally, there is an increase in energy expenditure as heat is lost in water evaporation from the skin. Finally, if, as may be the case, sepsis occurs a further metabolic strain is imposed on the body. It is therefore evident that the surface area and the degree of burns are the determining factors.

A large quantity of energy and nitrogen is required to cover the losses, which may continue for some time. In some instances, total parenteral nutrition is required before permitting enteral or normal oral intake.

PARENTERAL NUTRITION IN MAJOR TRAUMA

Metabolic response to trauma is described on p. 38. Tissue destruction and inflammatory exudate, containing protein rich fluid, are only two of the reasons for supplying a high calorie/protein diet. It is also necessary when the alimentary tract is unable to ingest or absorb nutrients due to direct involvement in the trauma, or when patients require artificial ventilation and/or develop infective complications.

PARENTERAL NUTRITION IN GASTROINTESTINAL DISORDERS

Among patients requiring parenteral feeding, there is a high proportion with gastrointestinal disorders. Not only those with obstructive

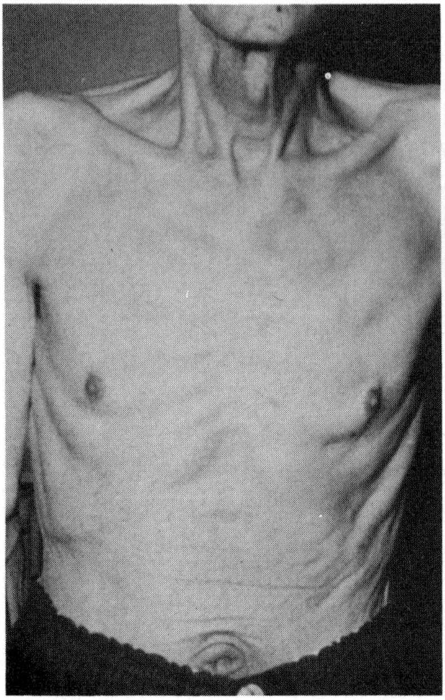

(*a*)

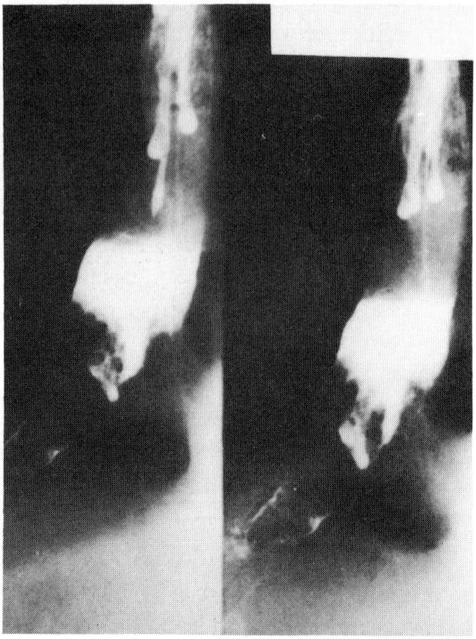

(*b*)

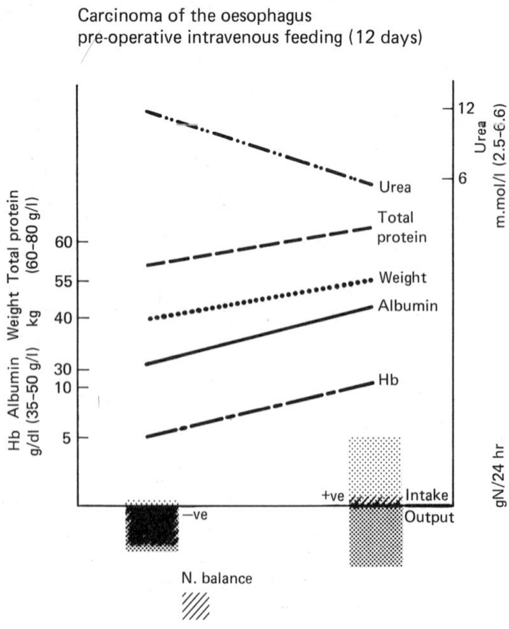
Carcinoma of the oesophagus
pre-operative intravenous feeding (12 days)
Hb g/dl
Albumin (35–50 g/l)
Weight kg
Total protein (60–80 g/l)
60
55
40
30
10
5
Urea m.mol/l (2.5–6.6)
12
6
Urea
Total protein
Weight
Albumin
Hb
gN/24 hr
+ve
–ve
Intake
Output
N. balance

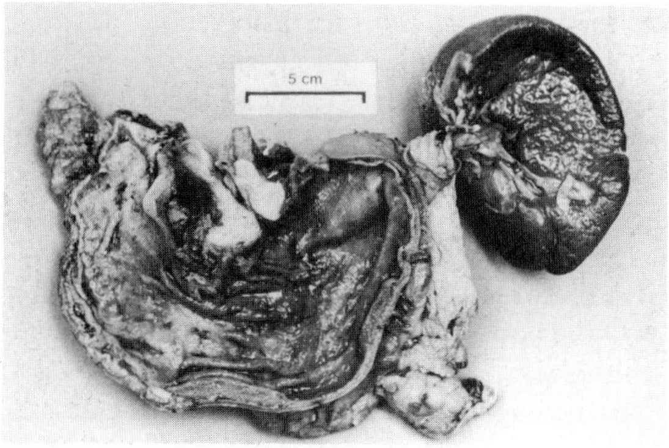

(*d*)

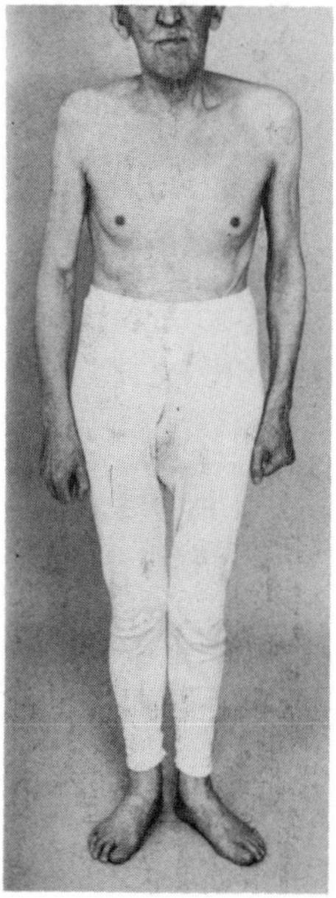

(*e*)

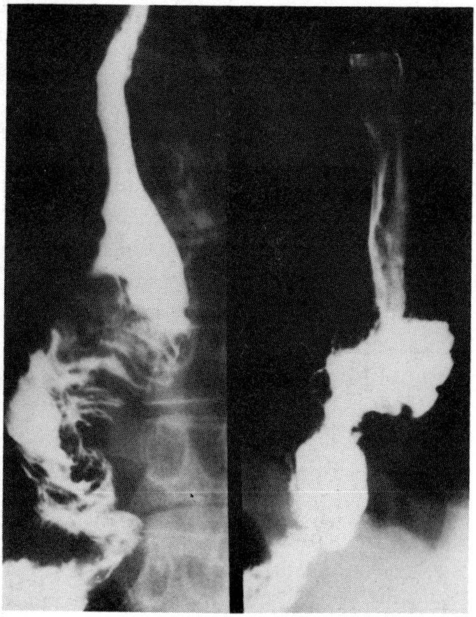

(*f*)

Fig. 3.1 (*a*) *Pre-operative photograph of patient with carcinoma of the oesophagus. Note the clinical features of malnutrition.* (*b*) *Barium swallow showing obstruction of the oesophagus with filling defect.* (*c*) *Some of the biochemical data of the patient on admission and after 12 days intravenous feeding (prior to surgery).* (*d*) *Resected specimen of the patient consisting of part of the oesophagus with tumour, the whole of the stomach, omentum and spleen.* (*e*) *Photograph of the patient 5 years after his operation.* (*f*) *Barium swallow of the patient 5 years after surgery showing the remainder of the oesophagus and jejunal loop.*

or neoplastic lesions are subjects for intravenous nutrition, but also patients with a variety of conditions characterized by the inability to absorb nutrients, or those affected by excessive loss of fluid rich in proteins and other nutrients.

In some cases (e.g. enteritis), profuse diarrhoea added to infection depletes the body of fluid and nutrients, as well as preventing absorption. In other conditions, exemplified by ulcerative colitis and regional ileitis, there may be lack of intake combined with protein and blood loss into the bowel. There may also be development of fistulae with resultant loss of fluid and electrolytes.

Intravenous feeding replaces the loss and provides the essential nutrients needed to improve the general condition of the patient and promote the healing of the bowel.

PARENTERAL NUTRITION IN HYPERCATABOLIC STATES

Hypercatabolic states are groups of metabolic conditions of differing aetiology in which there is an accelerated catabolism, with excessive protein breakdown and vast energy release in an attempt by the body to match the abnormally high metabolic demands. In effect, most medical and all surgical conditions are accompanied by some metabolic alterations with increased catabolism. Occasionally, however, the metabolic demands of a disease are such that the body burns itself up by its own fuel.

A surgical operation or multiple injury, when complicated by severe infection, brings about a hypercatabolic state. Extensive burns may be attended by a similar magnitude of catabolism. In some cases, the nitrogen output is increased to 3–4 times the normal level. In these circumstances, high calorie and protein intravenous feeding is the only treatment which is expected to succeed in restoring the metabolic equilibrium.

PARENTERAL NUTRITION IN SEVERE INFECTION

Parenteral nutrition is indicated in severe infection for a number of reasons:

1. There is a definite interaction between infection and malnutrition: undernourished individuals are immunologically deficient and may develop infection even by relatively harmless organisms.

2. In individuals with a chronic type of nutritional deficiency, infection can precipitate an acute and severe type of malnutrition.

3. Severe infections are accompanied by loss of appetite and decreased intake of nutrient.

4. Severe infections are attended by an increase in metabolism, with higher energy output, therefore requiring an increased level of energy and nitrogen intake.

While the nutritional therapy may not constitute the first-line treatment in many infections, which have to be treated by other means (i.e. antimicrobial agents), it is obvious that the malnourished individual is deprived of some of his defence mechanisms and must therefore be nutritionally supported. In some cases, the urgency of the situation and the magnitude of the metabolic disorders demand supplementary intravenous feeding or even total parenteral nutrition.

PARENTERAL NUTRITION AS AN ADJUNCT TO CHEMOTHERAPY

As discussed on p. 191, there are many reasons for cancer patients requiring nutritional support. In some there is a need for supplementary or total parenteral feeding.

Cancer cachexia presents with many clinical and biochemical features of malnutrition: commonly, extreme loss of weight, protein deficiencies and immunological incompetence are seen. It seems that in some cancer patients the severity of malnutrition (or malnutrition indices) parallels the extent of cancer expansion.

The submission of these patients to cancer chemotherapy is one of the difficult problems facing the oncologist, as well as all those involved in their management. Almost all chemotherapeutic agents (cytotoxic drugs) have an inhibitory effect on food intake, food absorption and utilization of nutrients, yet chemotherapy is mainly used in those with extensive and widespread disease who are already malnourished!

Among the many possible side-effects of chemotherapy, it is those related to the alimentary tract that are particularly disturbing, both metabolically and in a patient's quality of life. There is no doubt that chemotherapy suppresses the appetite and induces nausea and vomiting for a few days following intravenous injections. There is also ample evidence to suggest that, during this time, nutrition can be fully maintained by intravenous feeding (Copeland and Dudrick, 1978).

In spite of this, parenteral nutrition is not fully exploited in the UK. Nevertheless, it is being used by a few units with an advantageous effect both here and abroad.

12. Assessment of Nutritional Requirements and Selection of Nutrient Solutions

Assessment of nutritional requirements of a patient, together with the planning of the daily regime and selection of appropriate nutrient solutions, is considered one of the most important aspects of intravenous feeding. The assessment takes account of:

- The volume of water required.
- The amount of energy needed for metabolism.
- Protein as amino acids (nitrogen).
- Minerals, electrolytes, trace elements and vitamins.

Water

Total body water and the requirements needed to cover losses are described on p. 20. When assessing the water requirements of a patient, the following factors must be considered:

1. Normal water requirement to cover the physiological losses and to achieve water balance. This covers:

(a) Water loss by urine, e.g. the volume of urine necessary to eliminate waste and maintain haemostasis.
(b) Water needed to cover insensible perspiration, sweat, etc.

(c) Water to replace the volume lost by respiration (i.e. water contained in expired air).
(d) Water lost in faeces.

It is estimated that an adult takes in between 2500–2800 ml of water daily, and this amount achieves water equilibrium. If any of the components making up the water output are abnormally increased (e.g. diarrhoea), then the water intake has to be increased to compensate and achieve a new water balance equilibrium.

2. Extra water is necessary to cover the losses related to the disease.

It is worthwhile to recall that as part of the early response to trauma and injury, the body has a tendency to retain fluid (p. 39). Therefore, in the postoperative phase, the replacement of water is limited to the losses. The accuracy of a fluid balance chart cannot therefore be overstressed.

Taking into account the above factors, it is clear that the volume of water requirement varies greatly. For an average adult, with no great abnormal losses, an allowance of between 35–45 ml/kg is (in the authors' experience, and that revealed from literature) sufficient to cover requirements.

Energy requirements in intravenous feeding

The normal recommended intake of energy for a healthy individual is discussed on p. 32. In intravenous feeding, requirements are calculated and assessed on the basis of:

- The basic metabolic requirement.
- Energy needed for physical activity.
- Energy to cover the metabolism of the disease process.

Energy requirements for intravenous feeding are subject to variation because the basic metabolic requirements vary in different conditions and between individuals.

Basic metabolic requirements

Energy necessary for basal, or resting, metabolism of the subject is related to age, sex and bodyweight.

Passmore (1969) suggested the resting metabolic requirements for energy to be as shown in Table 3.1.

Table 3.1 Suggested metabolic requirements for energy (Passmore, 1969)

	kcal (MJ)/day
Age 0–1 years	400 (1.7)
Female aged 12–18 years	1400 (5.7)
Male aged 12–18 years	1700 (7.1)
Female over the age of 75 years	1100 (4.6)
Male over the age of 75 years	1350 (5.7)

The level of energy to cover the basal metabolic needs recommended by the Ministry of Agriculture Fisheries and Food Booklet (1979) for different ages and sex is shown in Table 3.2.

Close study of Table 3.2 shows little difference to that suggested by Passmore (Table 3.1). In effect, an adult requires about 1 kcal/min for his resting metabolism, which in practice is translated to 400–500 kcal for 8 hours sleep, i.e. the only time that there is a resting metabolism.

Table 3.2 Level of energy needed to cover basal metabolic requirements (Ministry of Agriculture, Fisheries and Food, 1979)

	Resting energy requirements	
	kcal (MJ)/day	*kcal (MJ)/kg/day*
Infant, 1-year-old	500 (2.1)	50 (0.21)
Child, 8-years-old	1000 (4.2)	40 (0.17)
Adult woman	1300 (5.4)	25 (0.1)
Adult man	1600 (6.7)	25 (0.1)

Energy allowance for physical activity

The value of this 'extra basal' requirement depends on the type of physical activity. There is also the energy for the specific dynamic action, that is energy used for various aspects of digestion and assimilation.

The sum total of energy requirements in healthy individuals is the amount which results in no longterm changes in weight. This amount is calculated on the basis of 8 hours each of sleep, work and recreational activity (Table 3.3).

The total recommended energy intake for healthy adults (DHSS recommendation) is indicated in Table 1.3, p. 35. Energy require-

Table 3.3 Energy requirements for an healthy individual leading a normal life

Designation	*Metabolic rate*	*kcal/min*	*kcal (MJ)*
8 hours sleep	Basal	1	530 (2.2)
8 hours work	Mild physical	1.4–2.5	870 (3.7)
8 hours recreational activity and some exercise	Moderate physical	1.4–5	1300 (5.8)
24 hours	Normal life	1–5	2700 (11.3)

ments are highest for men between the ages of 18–35 (2700 kcal/day) and lowest for women above the age of 75 years (1900 kcal/day).

In hospital patients and clinical situations, the assessment of an additional allowance of energy to cover physical activities (in the physiological sense) is difficult, and is based on experience and data recorded in experimental work. In physiological conditions, the total energy expenditure (i.e. basal and physical activity) has been calculated. This shows that the metabolic cost of standing and walking may introduce only a two- to three-fold increase in metabolism, but strenuous work may increase the metabolism by eight- to nine-fold.

For a patient in the ward, the calculation is based on the metabolic cost of sitting, standing and some walking, which for an average adult of 65 kg is calculated as in Table 3.4.

Table 3.4 Energy requirements of a patient (65 kg) in the hospital ward

	Average energy expenditure	
	kcal/min	*kJ/min*
Sitting	1.4	6
Standing	1.7	7
Walking slowly	3	13
Washing and dressing	3.5	15

Nutritional demands related to the illness

The allowance given to cover the extra metabolic cost, which is the consequence of a patient's illness, varies greatly depending on the type of the disease, its metabolic effects and any complications. Here, the assessment for an individual patient may meet with considerable difficulties. Short of direct or indirect metabolic studies (p. 4), which in everyday clinical situations are not feasible, there are two alternative ways to assess the metabolic requirements of the disease process.

1. It is possible to refer to nitrogen output and nitrogen balance and adjust the intake to achieve a positive nitrogen balance. As explained (p. 39), the metabolic response to injury is reflected in the nitrogen output which is estimated in the laboratory. The increase in the output of nitrogen, over and above that which is normally excreted, is due to catabolism of protein as a consequence of the injury. This amount of nitrogen, however, has to be matched with the amount of calories to be allocated. It has been suggested, and usually accepted, that 1 g of nitrogen in the metabolic process is matched to about 200 kcal of energy. (This is the ratio which appears to exist in healthy individuals on normal food intake.) By adopting this recommendation, and checking the adequacy of nitrogen intake by nitrogen balance studies, it is possible to obtain figures for energy intake.

2. For the last 25 years there has been a wealth of information about the metabolic requirements of individuals with specific conditions. It is therefore possible to refer to available data from published work to construct the energy requirements schedule for a patient. In patients receiving total parenteral nutrition, the basal energy requirement of 30 kcal (0.13 MJ)/kg bodyweight is suggested. This level has to be upgraded considerably in catabolic states. Even after an uncomplicated major surgical procedure, the energy requirement may be as high as 45–50 kcal/kg bodyweight (0.17–0.21 MJ/kg) (Table 3.5).

Table 3.5 Calorie and nitrogen allowance to achieve positive nitrogen balance in elective surgery

Authors	*gN/kg* b.w.	*kcal/kg* b.w.
Abbott *et al.* (1959)	0.20	35
Van Larsen and Brockner (1965)	0.24	32
Johnston *et al.* (1966)	0.16	33
Tweedle and Johnston (1971)	0.23	45
Johnston *et al.* (1972)	0.223	38
Moghissi and Teasdale (1980)	0.2–0.25	40–45

Protein, amino acids and nitrogen

The recommended protein intake for healthy adults is estimated at 55–68 g protein/day (p. 34) corresponding to about 10 g nitrogen/day. When assessing the requirements of protein for intravenous feeding, the following is considered:

1. Both essential and non-essential amino acids are required.
2. It is important to have a balanced ratio of energy to nitrogen allowance. This is suggested to be about 150–200 kcal of energy for 1 g of nitrogen.
3. Assessment must take account of :

(a) Normal requirements of the individual;
(b) Metabolic demands of the disease, which in turn is related to the magnitude of catabolism. In extensive injury and hypercatabolic states this amounts to a large increase in nitrogen losses, which has to be allowed for in the intake;
(c) The replacement of abnormal losses such as heavy discharges from surgical wounds, burns and fistulae.

In practice, the aim is to achieve nitrogen equilibrium. Table 3.5 gives some suggestions for nitrogen requirements for surgical patients. In hypercatabolic states the amount required is far above this.

Minerals, electrolytes and trace elements

The assessment of requirements for electrolytes is made by the addition of abnormal and increased losses (caused by the disease process) to the normal requirements (p. 26) that are included in intravenous feeding. Increased losses are determined by combined calculation of abnormal losses.

Overall requirements are gauged by daily adjustments guided by biochemical monitoring which, for the electrolytes, means daily testing. Table 3.6 gives suggested daily requirements for electrolytes and trace elements.

Vitamins

Both water and fat soluble vitamins are required in intravenous feeding. The amounts are calculated by normal and extra requirements in certain conditions.

Table 3.6 Suggested daily requirements for electrolytes and trace elements

	Allowances/kg bw in normal diet*	*Allowances/kg bw in parenteral nutrition*	*Authors*
Sodium	1–1.4 mmol/kg/day	2–3 mmol/kg/day with fat in diet (4.3 mmol/kg bw/day without fat) (1–1.4 mmol/kg bw/day with fat)	Dudrick *et al.*, 1969 (Wilmore *et al.*, 1969) (Grotte *et al.*, 1976)
Potassium	0.7–0.9 mmol/kg/day	7 mmol/g N (2 mmol/kg/day with fat) (3.9 mmol/kg/day without fat)	Lee, 1974 (Grotte, 1971) (Wilmore *et al.*, 1969)
Calcium		0.11 mmol/kg (0.5 mmol/kg)	(Grotte, 1971)
Magnesium	0.04 mmol/kg/24 hours	0.04 mmol/kg (1 mmol/kg)	Wretlind, 1972 (Wilmore *et al.*, 1969)
Iron	0.25–1.0 mol/kg	1 mol/kg (2 mol/kg)	Shils, 1972 (Fomon, 1967)
Manganese	0.1 mol/kg	0.6 mol/kg (0.7 mol/kg)	(Wilmore *et al.*, 1969)
Zinc	0.7 mol/kg	0.7 mol/kg (0.6 mol/kg)	Jacobson and Wester, 1977 (Wilmore *et al.*, 1969) RDA 1968
Copper	0.07 mol/kg	0.07 mol/kg (0.34 mol/kg)	Shils, 1972 (Wilmore *et al.*, 1969)
Iodine	0.015 mol/kg (0.04 mol/kg)	0.015 mol/kg (0.04 mol/kg)	
Phosphorus	0.15 mmol/kg	0.15 mmol/kg (1.5 mmol/kg) Should correspond to calcium intake	Recommended dietary allowance, 1968 (Ricour *et al.*, 1975)

( ) = for neonates and infants. * bw = bodyweight.

Table 3.7 Suggested allowances for vitamins in total parenteral nutrition

Vitamins	*Recommended daily allowance in adults*	*Allowance/kg bw** *in complete intravenous nutrition*
Thiamine	0.9–1.2 mg	0.02 mg
Riboflavin	1.3–1.7 mg	0.03 mg
Nicotinic acid	15–18 mg	0.2 mg
Folic acid	10–30 mg	3 μg
Vitamin B_{12}	about 3 mg	0.03 μg
Ascorbic acid	25–30 mg	0.5 mg
Vitamin A (retinol)	750 μg	10 μg
Vitamin D (cholecalciferol)	2.5 mg	0.04 mg
Vitamin K	about 2 mg	2 μg

* bw = bodyweight.

Some vitamins have a special role in the process of wound healing (e.g. vitamin C), which must be considered and accounted for. Table 3.7 gives the suggested allowance for vitamins in total parenteral nutrition.

NUTRIENT SOLUTIONS AND FORMULATION OF INTRAVENOUS REGIME

One of the most significant advances made in the clinical nutritional field in the last 25 years is the manufacturing and ready availability of suitable nutrient solutions for intravenous feeding.

The available intravenous feeding solutions in the UK are listed in Tables 3.8 and 3.9.

Energy sources

Carbohydrates, fat and alcohol are used as energy providers in intravenous feeding. Carbohydrates and alcohol are coupled with amino acid solutions, in varying concentration, to produce a nitrogen/calorie solution.

Table 3.8 Energy sources for intravenous feeding

Preparation		*Manufacturer*	*Constituents*	*pH*	*kcal (MJ)/l*
Intralipid 10%		KabiVitrum	Soya bean oil 50 g Glycerol 11 g	7.0	1100 (4.6)
Intralipid 20%		KabiVitrum	Soya bean oil 100 g Glycerol 11 g	7.0	2000 (8.4)
Glucoplex 1000		Geistlich	Carbohydrates, calories, electrolytes and trace metals	5–6	1000 (4.2)
Glucoplex 1600		Geistlich	Carbohydrates, calories, electrolytes and trace metals	5–6	1600 (6.8)
Glucose 5%	Polyfusor	Boots	Glucose	5–6	200 (0.85)
Glucose 10%	Polyfusor	Boots	Glucose	5–6	400 (1.7)
Glucose 20%	Polyfusor	Boots	Glucose	5–6	800 (3.4)
Glucose 40%	Polyfusor	Boots	Glucose	5–6	1600 (6.8)
Glucose 50%	Polyfusor	Boots	Glucose	5–6	2000 (8.4)

Carbohydrates

Dextrose, fructose and sorbitol are provided as separate solutions of differing strengths. These are also coupled with amino acid solutions and presented in one bottle, which provide a solution of energy and amino acid.

Alcohol

Ethanol is provided, coupled with amino acid solution.

Fat

At present the only available lipid preparation is *Intralipid*, an emulsion of fractionated soya bean oil which contains phospholipid and glycerol, giving a high caloric value in a small volume. It is of great practical use in a total parenteral nutrition programme.

Amino acid solutions

All available amino acid solutions contain, in varying proportions, essential and non-essential amino acids (Table 3.10). The majority are presented as a mixture of amino acids coupled with energy sources. Some mixtures contain sorbitol and/or ethanol, others contain fructose or glucose (Dextrose). There are also amino acid solutions without an additional energy source. Of particular interest is the amino acid in iso-osmolar solution (Perifusin).

Minerals, electrolytes and trace elements

Some of the available 'nutrient solutions' contain little, others no electrolytes whatsoever (Table 3.11).

Sodium chloride solution for infusion alone, or with dextrose, is however available and other electrolytes, notably potassium can be added to saline solution for infusion. Only recently, mixtures of electrolytes and trace elements have been made available containing calcium, magnesium, iron, zinc, manganese, copper, fluorine and iodine in appropriate proportions (Adamel of KabiVitrum).

Table 3.9 Amino acid solutions for parenteral nutrition

Preparations	*Manufacturers*	*Constituents*	*N Content g/l*	*Energy kcal (MJ)/l*	*pH*	*Osmolality*	*Availability ml*
Aminofusin L600	B.D.H. Pharmaceuticals (E. Merck)	L-amino acids Electrolytes Sorbitol	7.60	600 (2.5)	6.8	1300 mosm/kg	1000
Aminofusin L1000	B.D.H. Pharmaceuticals (E. Merck)	L-amino acids Electrolytes Sorbitol Ethanol	7.60	1000 (4.2)	6.8	2700 mosm/kg	1000
Aminofusin LForte	B.D.H. Pharmaceuticals (E. Merck)	L-amino acids Electrolytes Sorbitol Ethanol	30.40	800 (3.4)	5.5	1050 mosm/kg	500
Perifusin	B.D.H. Pharmaceuticals (E. Merck)	L-amino acids Electrolytes	5.00	132 (0.51)	7.1	3765 mosm/kg	1000
Aminoplex 5	Geistlich	L-amino acids Electrolytes Sorbitol Ethanol	5.00	1000 (4.2)	7.4	2415 mosm/kg	1000

Aminoplex 12	Geistlich	L-amino acids Electrolytes	12.44		7.4	830 mosm/kg	500 + 1000
Aminoplex 14	Geistlich	L-amino acids Electrolytes	13.40		5.5	875 mosm/kg	500
Freamine II	Boots Ltd	L-amino acids Electrolytes	12.50		6.6	850 mosm/kg	500
Synthamin 9	Travenol	L-amino acids Electrolytes	9.30		6.0	520 mosm/l	500
Synthamin 14	Travenol	L-amino acids Electrolytes	14.30		6.0	880 mosm/l	500
Synthamin 17	Travenol	L-amino acids Electrolytes	16.90		6.0	1060 mosm/l	500
Vamin fructose	KabiVitrum	L-amino acids Electrolytes Fructose	9.4	650 (2.9)	5.2	1260 mosm/kg of water	500
Vamin glucose	KabiVitrum	L-amino acids Electrolytes Glucose	9.4	650 (2.9)	5.2	1260 mosm/kg of water	100 + 500 + 1000
Vamin N	KabiVitrum	L-amino acids Electrolytes	9.4	250 (1.0)	5.2	700 mosm/kg	500 + 1000
Pluritene	Lipha Pharmaceuticals	L-amino acids	0.915 g/ per 100 ml	45 kcal/ 100 ml (0.2)	5.0		100 ml vial

Table 3.10 Amino acids in commercially available solutions

	Essential								Non-Essential										
	Leucine	*Isoleucine*	*Lysine*	*Threonine*	*Tryptophan*	*Methionine*	*Phenylalanine*	*Valine*	*Arginine*	*Histidine*	*Alanine*	*Glutamic acid*	*Proline*	*Glycine*	*Serine*	*Tyrosine*	*Cystine*	*Aspartic acid*	*% essential of total*
Aminofusin L600+L1000	+	+	+	+	+	+	+	+	+	+	+	+	+	+	–	–	–	–	26
Aminofusin LForte	+	+	+	+	+	+	+	+	+	+	+	+	+	+	–	–	–	–	27
Aminoplex 5	+	+	+	+	+	+	+	+	+	+	+	–	+	+	–	–	–	+	43
Aminoplex 12	+	+	+	+	+	+	+	+	+	+	+	+	+	+	+	–	–	+	46
Aminoplex 14	+	+	+	+	+	+	+	+	+	+	+	–	+	+	–	–	–	–	45
Freamine 2	+	+	+	+	+	+	+	+	+	+	+	–	+	+	+	–	+	–	48
Synthamin 9, 14+17	+	+	+	+	+	+	+	+	+	+	+	–	+	+	–	+	–	–	40
Vamin glucose+fructose	+	+	+	+	+	+	+	+	+	+	+	+	+	+	+	+	+	+	41
Perifusin	+	+	+	+	+	+	+	+	+	+	+	+	+	+	–	–	–	–	26

Table 3.11 Minerals and vitamins in nutrient solutions for parenteral feeding

	mmols							mg				
Preparations	Na^{+}	K^{+}	Mg^{++}	Ca^{++}	Cl^{-}	PO_4^{+++}	*Acetate*	*Vitamin C*	*Inositol*	*Nicotinamide*	*Pyridoxine*	*Riboflavine*
Aminofusin L600	+	+	+	−	+	−	+	+	+	+	+	+
Aminofusin L1000	+	+	+	−	+	−	+	+	+	+	+	+
Aminofusin LForte	+	+	+	−	+	−	+	−	+	+	+	+
Aminoplex 5	+	+	−	−	+	−	−	−	−	+	+	−
Aminoplex 12	+	+	+	−	+	−	+	−	−	−	−	−
Aminoplex 14	+	+	−	−	+	−	−	−	−	+	+	−
Freamine II	+	−	−	−	−	+	−	−	−	−	−	−
Perifusin	+	+	+	−	+	−	+	−	−	−	−	−
Synthamin 9	+	+	+	−	+	+	+	−	−	−	−	−
Synthamin 14	+	+	+	−	+	+	+	−	−	−	−	−
Synthamin 17	+	+	+	−	+	+	+	−	−	−	−	−
Vamin N	+	+	+	+	+	−	−	−	−	−	−	−
Vamin fructose	+	+	+	+	+	−	−	−	−	−	−	−
Vamin glucose	+	+	+	+	+	−	−	−	−	−	−	−

Vitamins

Hydrosoluble and liposoluble (fat soluble) vitamins are now available and used as additives. The water soluble vitamins are added to glucose solutions, and fat soluble vitamin preparations are added to lipid solution (Intralipid).

PRESCRIBING A REGIME FOR INTRAVENOUS FEEDING

The basic principle of arranging a regime is to first assess the nutritional requirements of a particular patient in terms of calorie and nitrogen and the volume of water intake, then to select from the available nutrient solutions those which adequately cover those requirements. Electrolytes, vitamins and trace elements are given as for 'normal requirements', and additional amounts are added according to the results of regular biochemical monitoring.

In practice, however, certain additional points are considered:

1. Some adjustments in the diet are inevitable during the course of intravenous therapy, in spite of all the care taken to formulate a regime based on a comprehensive assessment. This is particularly important with regard to water and electrolytes, particularly sodium and potassium. In effect, all parenteral nutrition solutions contain insufficient amounts of electrolytes, and these must therefore be added.

2. The optimum mixture of energy providers within a regime may alter in specific circumstances. Nevertheless, lipid solutions have several distinct advantages. For a small infusion volume, fat provides a high level of energy. In fact, energy derived from fat can form up to 60–80% of the total energy (Peaston, 1966; Stell, 1970). Many plan a regime in which fat provides 40–50% of total energy.

3. The optimum ratio of energy (kcal) to nitrogen (g) varies from case to case, but it is advisable to design the regime on the basis of the ratio of 150–200 kcal to 1 g of nitrogen.

4. Alcohol (ethanol) is used as a source of energy, but, to prevent inebriation, the rate of infusion is adjusted to dispense no more than 10 g/h of ethanol.

5. It is sound practice to administer vitamins and trace elements daily.

6. Attention is paid to the overall osmolar load—at any rate hypertonic solutions are administered slowly (Table 3.9).

7. Attention is also paid to acid base balance. Many of the solutions for intravenous infusion are acidic. In addition, the products of metabolism are acidic rather than alkaline. Critically-ill patients, in particular, have difficulty in maintaining their acid base balance and need careful monitoring. If necessary, the pH is adjusted by infusion of the appropriate solutions.

Summary of daily regime

The following data is based on the authors' experience and others:

Water	35–45 ml/kg bodyweight (bw): monitor—alter as required
Minerals	
Sodium	1–1.5 mmol/kg bw: monitor—alter
Potassium	1 mmol/kg bw: monitor
Others (trace elements)	Add daily
Energy	30–50 or more kcal/kg bw according to metabolic rate (40–50% fat)
Nitrogen (Amino acid)	0.11–0.25 or more g/kg bw according to catabolism
Vitamins	Add daily

- Pay attention to osmolality: administer slowly hyperosmolar solutions.
- Pay attention to acid base balance.

13. Delivery of Nutrient Solutions to Patients

Intravenous feeding is achieved by the delivery of nutrients into the blood stream. When intravenous feeding is used for long periods, and remains the sole method of nutrition, its management should be undertaken by a nutritional team that has the technical knowledge and full laboratory facilities to hand. However, the majority of patients require intravenous feeding for limited periods of 2–3 weeks and are usually accommodated in medical or surgical wards of a district general hospital. One of the most important advances made in intravenous feeding is the development of relatively simple, and yet safe, methods of delivering infusion which allows this type of feeding to be undertaken in the general ward. Therefore it is essential that both medical and nursing staff understand the principles, and their application, in order to undertake intravenous feeding as part of the general management of patients. For this reason, technical aspects of intravenous feeding need to be familiar to nurses in medical and surgical wards. This is described under the headings of circulatory access and infusion equipment.

CIRCULATORY ACCESS

A well-placed intravenous catheter is an essential requirement for intravenous feeding. Theoretically, solutions for intravenous infusion are delivered through any vein, but in practice, the modes of delivery may be as follows:

1. Peripheral vein cannulation.
2. Central vein catheterization:

   (a) direct central vein catheterization;
   (b) central vein catheterization via a peripheral vein.

In each case the vein is entered by percutaneous puncture or cut-down technique.

Peripheral vein cannulation

This route (Fig. 3.2) is generally unsuitable for parenteral feeding as the amino acid and hypertonic sugar solutions, in particular, irritate the veins and cause thrombophlebitis. If this route is used for total parenteral nutrition, the site is changed every 24–48 hours. However, some lipids and isotonic amino acids may be infused into a peripheral vein for longer periods. The technique is useful in the ward for emergency placement of a short cannula.

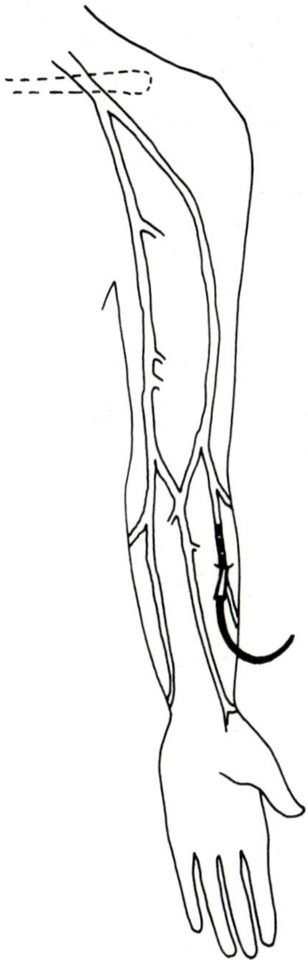

Fig. 3.2 Peripheral vein cannulation.

Insertion of peripheral vein cannula

A large vein is selected. Lower limb veins are not used because this adds to the patient's immobility and creates a higher risk of complications. When a peripheral vein is cannulated for intravenous nutrition, rigorous antiseptic precautions are observed. The skin is cleaned thoroughly by prolonged rubbing, using an antiseptic solution (Hibitane in spirit or alcoholic povidone-iodine) which is allowed to dry before venapuncture is carried out. Although proper fixation of the cannula is essential to avoid extrusion of the cannula or extravasation of nutrients, the fixation should not exclude examination of the site of the catheter. Any additional splints, bandages, etc., make it difficult to inspect the site of insertion regularly, and are not required if the cannula is correctly placed well away from any joints. Transparent, adhesive semi-occlusive dressings (e.g. Op-Site) allow securing of the cannula and ready observation. The site of insertion is sometimes dressed with a sterile gauze swab which is easily removed and replaced aseptically to allow inspection.

There are a variety of short intravenous cannulae for percutaneous puncture (Table 3.12), which contain a needle or a fine trocar within a plastic cannula.

Cut-down technique for cannulation of peripheral vein

Occasionally it is necessary to cut-down into a peripheral vein for cannulation. This is now rarely practised for insertion of a short cannula, but may be employed for catheterization with a long catheter passed via a peripheral vein into a central vein (e.g. from one of the antecubital veins into the superior vena cava).

Central vein catheterization

This usually means the use of the inferior or the superior vena cava. The inferior vena cava is not favoured, as it is not easily reached percutaneously and prevents active mobilization of the patient. The superior vena cava is generally used for intravenous feeding. Several techniques are employed to place the catheter. Figure 3.3a shows points of insertion for central venous catheterization.

Direct central vein catheterization

This is achieved by percutaneous puncture of the external jugular, internal jugular or subclavian vein, which is approached by infra-clavicular puncture (Fig. 3.3b). Alternatively, a cut-down technique is used to approach the vein surgically. Whether the vein is entered by percutaneous puncture, or by incision and cut-down technique, a length of the catheter near the 'hub', or giving set end, may be placed in a subcutaneous tunnel to protect the immediate entry site of the vein from contamination and reduce the risk of infection.

A central vein catheter may be used for a considerable length of time without any complications, providing it is well and properly

Table 3.12 Intravenous cannulae

Designation	Manufacturer	Material		Specific features
Cathlon	Criticon	Teflon	(N)	Metal hub and luer lock
Jelco	Criticon	Teflon	(N)	Plastic hub and luer lock
Surflo	Cory Bros.	Siliconized needle		Plastic hub and luer lock Coloured wings. Coding
Medicut	Argyle	Polypropylene	(N)	Plastuc hub and luer lock Matching syringe for easy insertion and provided in a plastic tube—colour-coded according to diameter
Medicut T	Argyle	Teflon	(N)	With/without syringe
I.V. Cannula	Portex	Nylon	(N)	Plastic luer lock or record mount with wing/butterly. Packed in carton
Angiocath	Deseret	Teflon	(N)	Radio-opaque. Luer lock adaptor. In plastic container Colour-coded wing according to gauge
Intraflon 2	Vygon	Teflon	(N)/(C)	There are long and short cannulae. Plastic hub and luer lock. Flexible wing
Intranule	Vygon	Polypropylene		Cannula mounted on a trocar. Plastic hub and wing

(N) = Needle inside cannula
(C) = Cannula inside needle

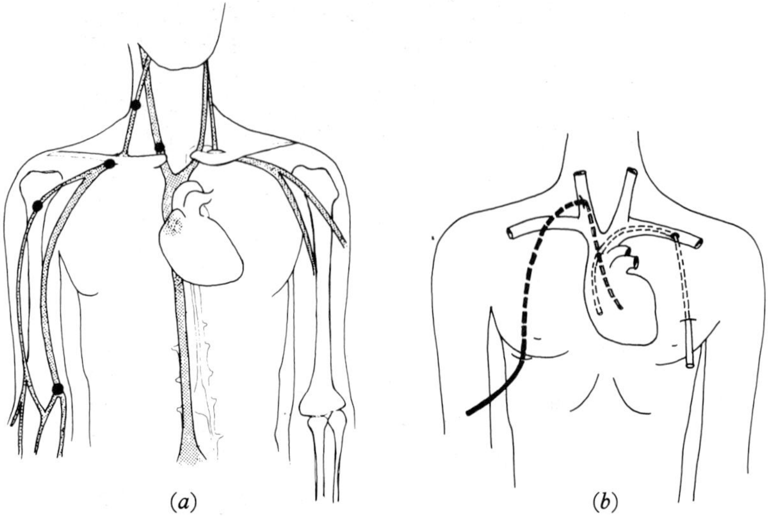

(*a*) (*b*)

Fig. 3.3 (*a*) *Points of insertion for central venous catheterization* (*from above downwards*)*: 1. External jugular vein; 2. Internal jugular vein; 3. Subclavian vein* (*direct insertion*)*; 4. Cephalic vein; 5. Basilic vein.* (*b*) *Shows percutaneous puncture of left subclavian and right internal jugular vein* (*with subcutaneous tunnelling*).

placed and carefully managed. General guidelines for central vein catheterization are:

1. Insertion of catheter using percutaneous technique is carried out in the operating theatre, intensive care unit (ICU), clinical room of the ward, or, if absolutely necessary, in the ward.

2. The cut-down technique is best carried out in the ICU or operating theatre.

3. Usually, catheters are placed under local anaesthesia. However, if a patient is to receive general anaesthesia for other reasons (such as endoscopy), the catheter is inserted at the same time.

4. Whether a cut-down or a percutaneous technique is used for establishing the intravenous infusion, the procedure is considered as a surgical operation and strict, aseptic techniques must therefore be observed.

5. In all cases the position of the catheter in a central vein is checked radiologically (Fig. 3.4).

The nutrient solutions are particularly favourable for the culture of micro-organisms, and the catheter itself forms an easy port of entry

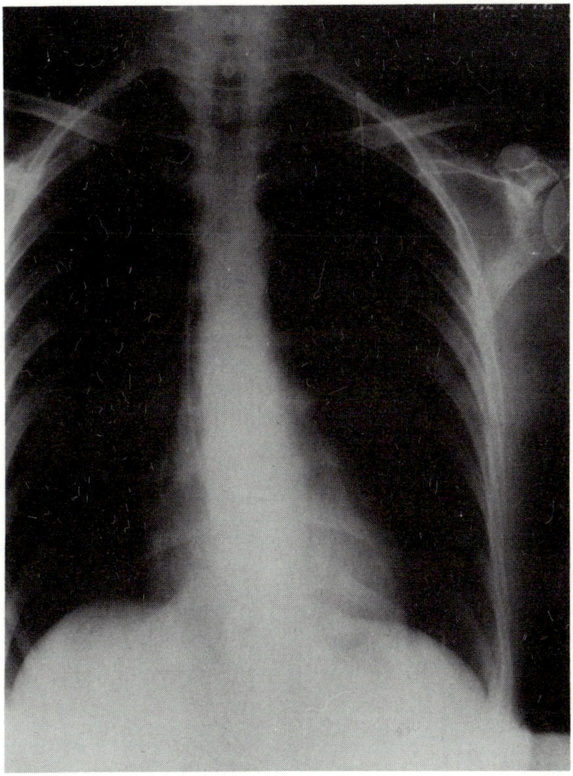

Fig. 3.4 Correct position of the catheter. In this case in the right atrium.

for the introduction and spread of organisms within the body. In order to minimize this risk, the patient's skin is cleaned by scrubbing it thoroughly with an antiseptic solution (such as alcoholic povidone-iodine, or Hibitane in spirit). This also cleans the hairs on the skin, although they may need to be shaved to facilitate insertion and securing of the cannula/catheter. There is some evidence that shaving results in microabrasions of the skin and methods of skin preparation before catheter insertion require further study. The operator thoroughly washes hands and forearms with an antiseptic detergent and wears a gown, mask and sterile gloves. When carrying out the procedure the following is applicable.

The area surrounding the insertion site is draped with sterile towels.

Once the catheter is inserted, it is fixed to the skin (usually by stitches), sprayed with polybactrin and a dressing applied.

The dressing is usually semi-permeable transparent film (e.g. Op-Site) to allow regular observation of the site.

The infusion set is secured in such a way as to allow ready access for management.

Suggested equipment for percutaneous puncture of the subclavian vein is shown in Fig. 3.5.

Cut-down technique for catheterization of central vein

In this technique, a surgical cut-down is made over a large vein (usually in the neck) and a catheter is introduced directly into the vein. The external or internal jugular vein is the usual site.

When the external jugular vein is to be catheterized, it is first exposed and then two lengths of catgut (0000 chromic) are passed around it. The distal (that is the cephalic) end of the vein is tied off, and the proximal end left untied but elevated to stop the backward flow of blood. An incision is made over the dissected vein between the two pieces of catgut and the catheter is carefully introduced, aiming to place its tip to lie in the superior vena cava or right atrium. The proximal end of the catgut is then tied around the proximal part of the vein, with the catheter fitted snugly within it. Usually, when the cut-down technique of catheterization is used, the catheter end is tunnelled subcutaneously for some distance and brought out of a separate skin incision over the chest wall (p. 110). The catheter is connected to the infusion set. The original neck incision is then closed, and the catheter fixed to the skin (Fig. 3.6).

In some cases, the external jugular vein may prove difficult to catheterize. When the internal jugular vein is the chosen vein for catheterization, a purse string suture is inserted loosely over the site of the introduction into the internal jugular vein, using 00000 silk or prolene. The catheter is introduced into the vein through the purse string suture, which is then tightened and tied around the catheter.

Suggested equipment for the cut-down technique of central venous catheterization is shown in Figs 3.7a,b.

Subcutaneous tunnelling of the catheter

For some time now the subcutaneous tunnelling of a length of the intravenous catheter, just distal to its point of entry into the vein, has

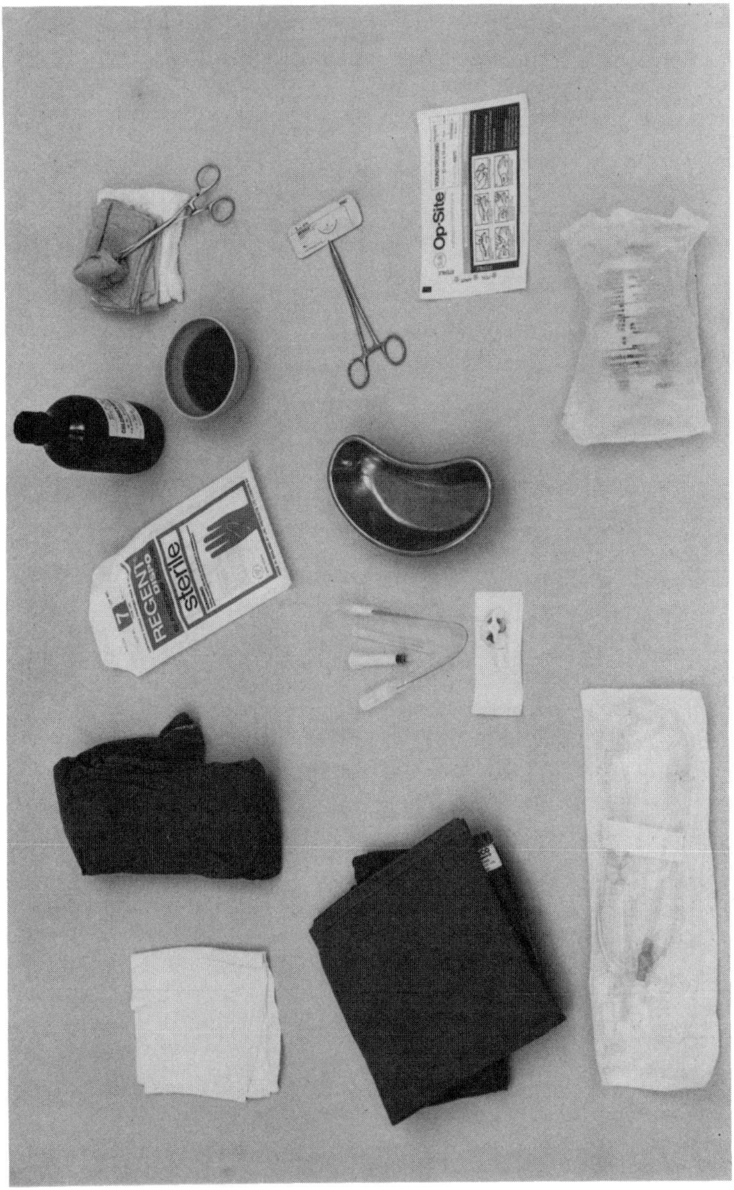

Fig. 3·5 Equipment for insertion of central venous catheter by percutaneous method. Top row *(from left to right): sterile hand towel, sterile gown, sterile gloves, antiseptic solution and gallipot, swab and swab holder.* Middle row *(from left to right): sterile towel, intravenous catheter syringe and cannula with inside needle (catheter kit), two-way tap, kidney dish, skin suture and needle holder, Op-Site dressing.* Bottom row *(from left to right): infusion system, bland intravenous solution.*

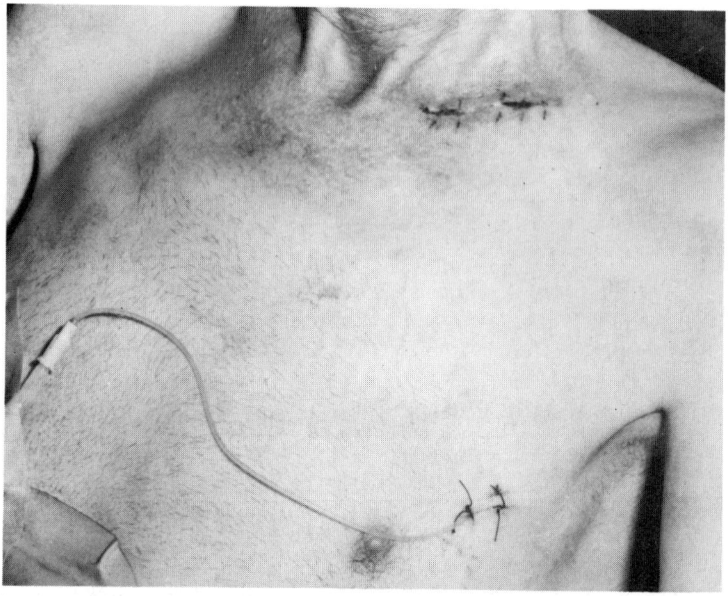

Fig. 3.6 Shows the central venous catheterization via external jugular vein using the cut-down technique and subcutaneous tunnelling.

been advocated. The idea was introduced by Scribner *et al.* (1970) and later successfully applied by others for subclavian and other central venous catheterization for intravenous nutrition.

The aim of the method is:

- To separate the point of entry of the catheter into the vein from its point of entry into the skin, thereby preventing movement of the catheter in and out of the vein.
- To prevent a 'possibly contaminated' section of the catheter, i.e. its exposed end, transmitting infection into the vein due to its proximity.
- To have some length of the catheter between its exposed part and the section in the vein, surrounded by 'biological' tissues which could limit the spread of infection to the vein.

The technique consists of:

1. Making a skin incision on the chest wall some distance away from the entry of the catheter into the vein (be it by percutaneous puncture or cut-down).

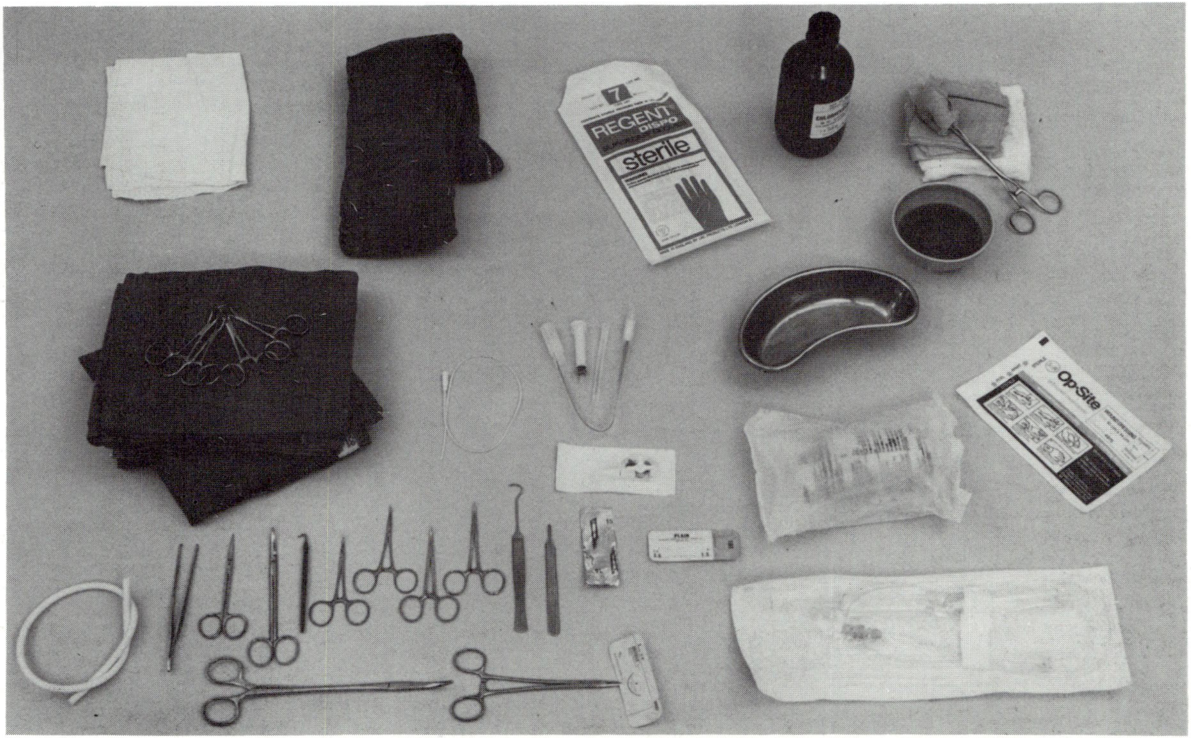

Fig. 3.7 (*a*) *Suggested equipment for insertion of central venous catheter by cut-down technique.* Top row (*from left to right*) *: sterile hand towel, sterile gown, sterile gloves, antiseptic solution, gallipot for same, swab and swab holder.* Middle row (*from left to right*) *: sterile towel and towel clips, intravenous catheter (or intravenous catheter kit consisting of catheter syringe and cannula with inside needle), two way tap, kidney dish, intravenous solution, Op-Site dressing.* Bottom row (*from left to right*) *: length of tubing for subcutaneous tunnelling (see p. 113); instruments for cut down including surgical blade, chromic catgut, needle holder with skin stitch, infusion system.*

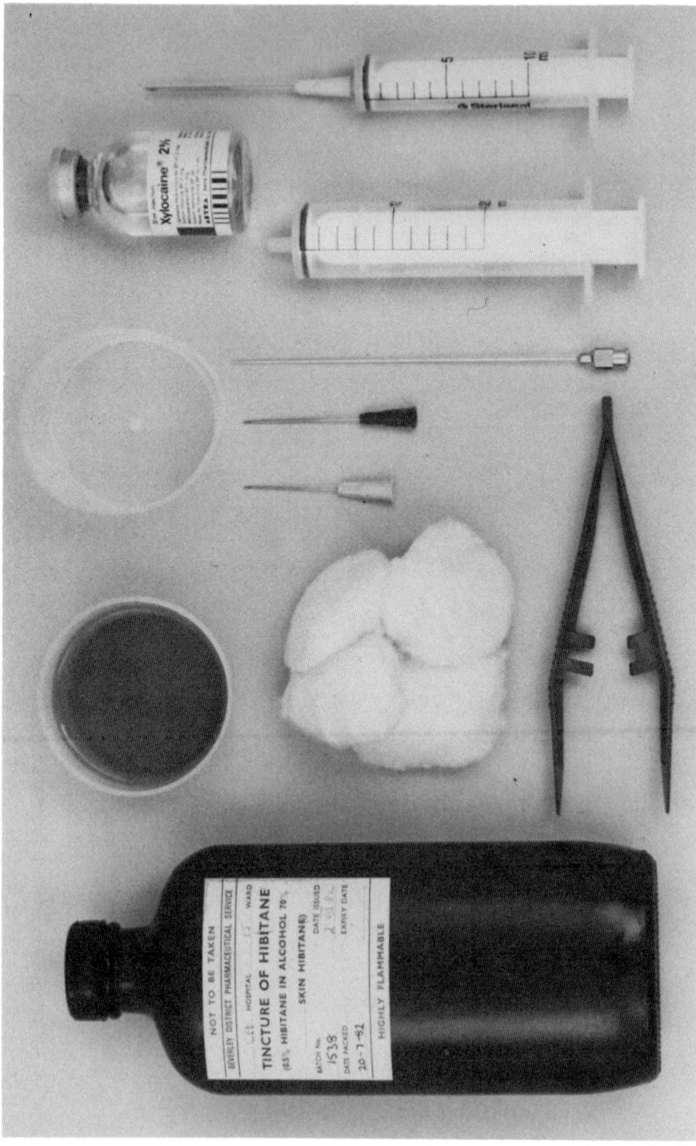

Fig. 3.7 (b) Suggested local anaesthetic equipment for intravenous catheterization.

2. A subcutaneous tunnel is made between the skin incision and the point of entry of the catheter into the vein. This is done by a long Roberts', or cholecystectomy, forceps.

3. A urinary catheter, such as a Jacques' catheter, or a length of plastic tubing of appropriate diameter, is then passed through the tunnel to the site of the insertion of the intravenous catheter.

4. The hub end of the intravenous catheter is then fed into the tube, which is withdrawn through the skin incision to bring the end of the intravenous catheter (which is now passing within the subcutaneous tunnel) out of the skin.

5. The end of the catheter is then connected to a giving set and fixed by stitches to the skin (Fig. 3.6).

Central vein catheterization via peripheral vein

This procedure (Fig. 3.8) consists of the placement of a long catheter through a peripheral vein and guided to a central vein, or superior vena cava and right atrium. An antecubital vein is usually used and the catheter is introduced percutaneously, or by a cut-down technique, and then advanced into the vein. The method is particularly suitable in emergency cases when the catheter has to be inserted in the ward.

Equipment for insertion of central vein catheter

The varying techniques of catheter placement, as well as different

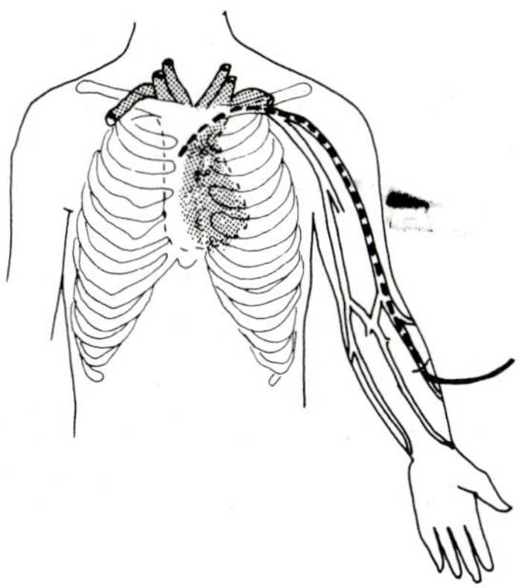

Fig. 3.8 Central venous catheterization via peripheral vein.

operators, may require different sets of equipment for inserting the infusion catheter. Nevertheless, the equipment is basically the same, albeit with minor variations, irrespective of what individual technique is used.

As a guideline, however, two sets of equipment are illustrated in Figs 3.4; 3.7a,b; one for the placement of the catheter by percutaneous technique as into the subclavian vein, and the other for the surgical cut-down technique with subcutaneous tunnelling of the catheter.

Following insertion of the catheter

By whichever method the central venous catheter is placed, it is always secured to the skin (usually by a skin stitch). The end is then connected to a two-way tap. An antibiotic spray is then applied and the whole area, except the very end of the catheter and the two-way tap, is covered by a sterile, semi-permeable, transparent, adhesive sheet such as Op-Site. In some instances, a short length of additional steriplastic catheter, with connectors at both ends, may be conveniently interposed between the intravenous catheter, and the two-way tap and infusion giving set. Figure 3.9 illustrates fixation and dressing of the central venous catheter.

INFUSION EQUIPMENT FOR INTRAVENOUS FEEDING

Intravenous nutrition depends on the delivery of the nutrients into the blood stream via the venous system. Besides the nutrient solution, which constitutes the 'feed', an infusion giving set and a suitable catheter for placement in the vein is required (Fig. 3.10). In addition, there are other accessory devices, e.g. filters, mini pumps, flow regulators, etc.

Cannulae and catheters for intravenous feeding

The present status of intravenous feeding has been reached by development in many directions, one of which is the design and manufacture of suitable intravenous cannulae and catheters. In this

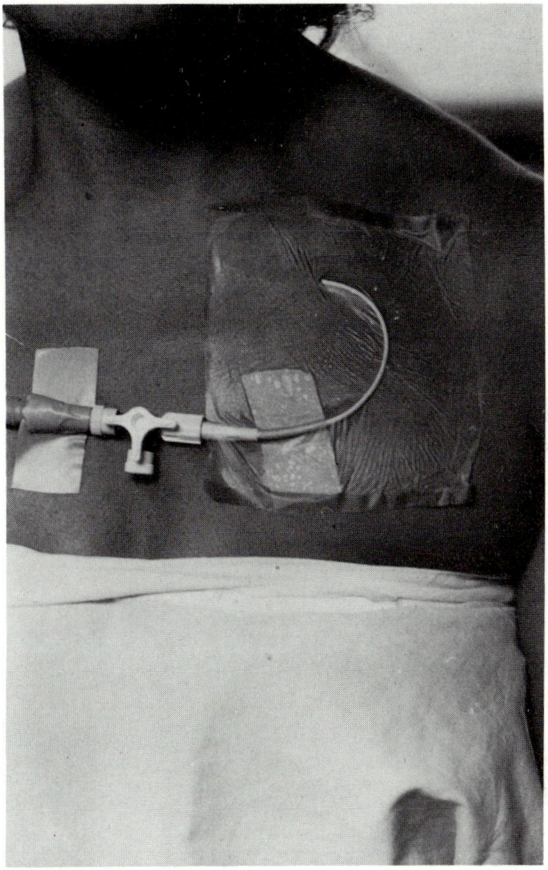

Fig. 3.9 Fixation of central venous catheter with two-way tap and Op-Site dressing. Note the Op-Site covers part of the hub, leaving the end free to connect with the two-way tap.

book, cannula refers to a short catheter (up to 5 cm) and to a longer intravenous infusion tube. Much effort has been made, and considerable resources allocated, to produce catheters which permit long periods of total parenteral nutrition with minimal risk. Putting aside the adventurous age of experimentation (or rather exploration), and the use of such devices as a 'goose quill' as a cannula for administration of infusions, the early intravenous devices were made of metal. As recently as the 1950s, needles and metal cannulae were the only form of apparatus in common use for infusion of intravenous fluids.

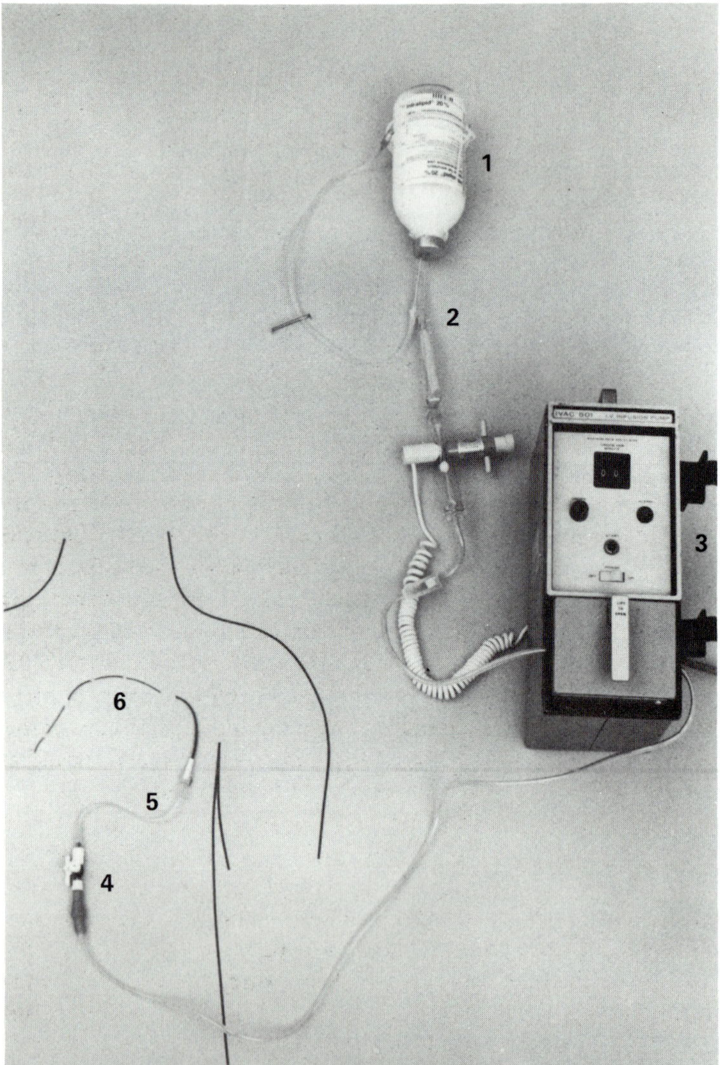

Fig. 3.10 Infusion equipment for parenteral feeding (with pump). 1. Nutrient bottle; 2. Infusion system (drip set); 3. Flow regulator (Ivac gravity); 4. Two-way tap; 5. Extension tube; 6. Catheter shown diagrammatically to enter superior vena cava.

There are now a variety of suitable cannulae and catheters available for intravenous feeding—polypropylene, polyethylene, teflon and silicone have replaced metal cannulae and, by the very nature of their flexibility, catheters of variable length are available for use in intravenous catheterization by any technique and in any circumstances.

While the selection of an intravenous feeding catheter is a matter of preference, and the choice of the clinician inserting it, the nursing staff, supply department of the hospital and the pharmacist are also involved in the provision of them. It is therefore useful to have some knowledge of the existing cannulae and catheters and their characteristics. Cannulae generally remain for short periods in a peripheral vein or, as can be seen on p. 124, are used as a means of introduction for a longer intravenous catheter.

Catheters are expected to remain within a vein for long or indefinite periods. A suitable catheter is one which has the following properties:

1. Flexibility. It is believed that the stiffer the catheter (and that is related to the material used in its manufacture), the more risk there is of internal damage to the vein and consequent phlebitis. Therefore, catheters made of silicone rubber are probably safest as they are more flexible than those of polyethylene or nylon. However, many catheters made of other materials are consistently used by many without complications. Other factors, such as the method and route of placement, and the position of the catheter tip, are important in the causation of phlebitis. The material used for making the catheter must be chemically inert so that it does not disintegrate or be affected by blood. It must also be non-reactive to body fluid.
2. The catheter must not break.
3. The catheter 'hub' and 'adaptors' must not crack or break.
4. The catheter for central venous positioning must be radio-opaque and/or have an x-ray detectable band.
5. There must not be any great discrepancy between the external and internal diameter of the catheter. In other words, the catheter must be thin yet strong, and flexible but not breakable.
6. The catheter alone, or as part of the set or the 'kit', must allow easy placement and fixation. After insertion, the catheter must not be in direct contact with the needle (p. 124).

An ideal catheter is one that allows a long or indefinite period of trouble-free total parenteral nutrition. Some examples are discussed below.

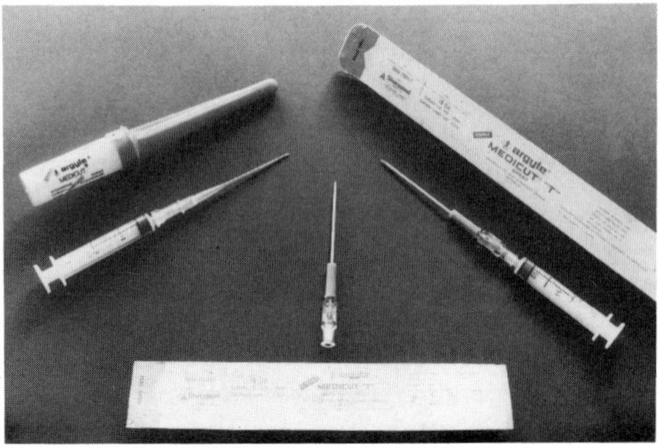

Fig. 3.11 Argyle medicut short cannula. Top left: *Argyle medicut short cannula.* Top right: *as above with provision of a long catheter.*

Cannulae

These are short fine tubes with a diameter range of about 1–3.5 mm and a length of 4–5 cm. They contain a needle which is slightly longer and of a smaller diameter. Consequently, the needle is accommodated within the cannula and its tip is bare of the plastic, i.e. the cannula is outside the needle. These cannulae are suitable for peripheral vein puncture and infusion. In practice the needle, which is covered by its plastic cannula and attached to a syringe, is introduced into the vein. The needle is then removed and the cannula advanced further into the vein, connected to the giving set and fixed to the skin in its desired position. An example is the Medicut Intravenous cannula (manufactured by Argyle, Fig. 3.11). Table 3.12 presents some of the currently available cannulae in the UK.

Intravenous catheters

These are long flexible plastic tubes which are usually introduced into a central vein. In many cases the catheter is to remain *in situ* for more than a few days and has to provide a channel of delivery for the high calorie and protein nutrients of high osmolality.

Table 3.13 gives the characteristics of some of the catheters available in the UK. These are principally of three kinds:

1. Catheter inside the needle.
2. Catheter with inside stilette.
3. Catheter without needle.

Table 3.13 Catheters for intravenous feeding

Designation	*Manufacturer*	*Material*	*Specific features*
Intramedicut	Argyle	Polypropylene (XR)	Needle inside cannula and catheter to be introduced through the cannula. A syringe is provided for easy insertion. The catheter is provided as a 'kit'
Cafafix MT	Braun	Polyethylene (XR)	Set comprises of needle, cannula and syringe. A plastic sheath holds the catheter
E.Z. Cath	Deseret	Teflon (XR)	Catheter sleeve provided. Special individual colour-coded pack
I.V. Catheter	Portex	Nylon (XR)	Needle inside cannula then a catheter to go through cannula. With/without wing. 30–76 cm
Gentrasil	Vicra (Travenol)	Silicone (XR)	Needle inside a cannula and catheter to be introduced through the cannula. Set comprising of catheter and accessories provided
Catheter-Stericath	Vygon	Polyethylene (XR)	Catheter passing inside the needle. A guard is provided to protect the catheter from the needle after insertion of the catheter
Leader Cath	Vygon	Polyethylene (XR)	Set comprises of syringe, needle, guide wire and catheter (Seldingers technique). Available in a wide range of lengths and sizes
Long line	Vygon	Polyethylene (XR)	Set comprises of needle, cannula and long catheter with a plastic sleeve. Available in 3 lengths and 3 diameters. With locking device
Nutricath	Vygon	Silicone (XR)	Stilett and Teflon introducer. Catheters of 35–60 cm

XR = radiopaque.

Catheter inside the needle. In these the venapuncture is made by the needle, and the catheter pushed through it and placed through the needle into the vein. The needle is then withdrawn, leaving the catheter in the vein. The catheter is advanced further into the vein to the desired position. The needle surrounding the end of the catheter is fixed over a 'guard', which is provided. Because of the particular danger of the catheter being severed by the needle, even when it is well protected by the guard, the use of this particular type of catheter has now been generally discontinued. Instead, based on the same principles, catheters are placed through a short cannula, which is first introduced into the vein. These catheter sets are made up of a short cannula with an inside needle attached to a syringe, and a long catheter which fits into the short cannula.

The needle and the cannula are first introduced into the vein, and the needle withdrawn, leaving the short cannula in the vessel. The long catheter is now introduced through the cannula and advanced into the desired position. When this is achieved, the short cannula is withdrawn from the vein and surrounds the catheter. The catheter and the cannula are fixed to the skin and the end of the catheter is connected to the drip set (e.g. Argyle Intramedicut Catheter Kit (Fig. 3.12a) and Vygon Long Line (Fig. 3.12b).

Catheter with inside stilette. These are long catheters with a stilette inside. The latter continues as a flexible wire which runs inside the whole length of the catheter. The stilette, surrounded by the catheter, is introduced into the vein and partly withdrawn, leaving the catheter which is advanced to its required position in the vein (e.g. E.Z. Catheter manufactured by Deseret). The stilette introducer is then completely removed and the catheter connected to the giving set and fixed to the skin.

Catheters without needle. These are of teflon or silicone fine bore tubing and are used for intravenous infusions when the surgical cut-down method is used. The vein is first exposed surgically and incised. The catheter is then introduced and positioned. There are still some catheters available for the cut-down technique. However, any of the other catheters designed for percutaneous placement (Table 3.13) may be used for intravenous infusion established by the cut-down technique, by simply using the 'catheter part' alone (without the needle) and the cannula, which are parts of the 'kit'.

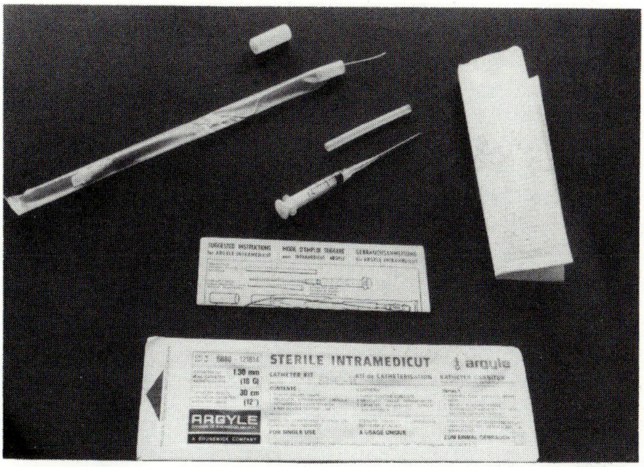

(*a*)

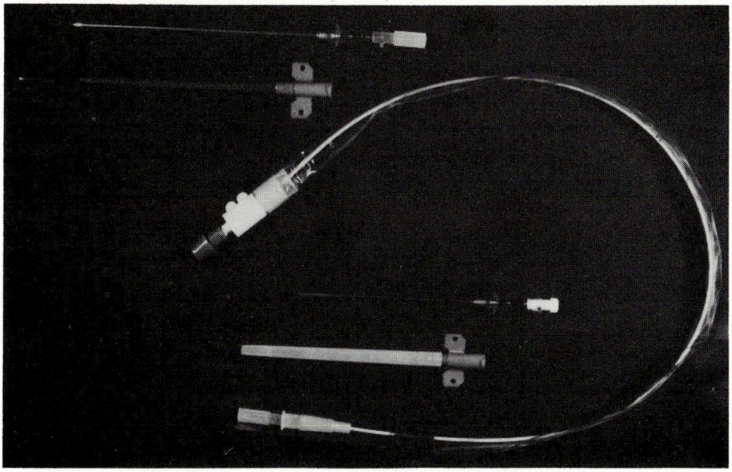

(*b*)

Fig. 3.12 (*a*) *Argyle intramedicut kit for catheterization of a central vein using percutaneous technique.* (*b*) *Vygon long-line used for central venous catheterization.*

Infusion sets and containers

There are now several types of infusion set for intravenous infusion. All sets are made of plastic, pre-packed and sterilized ready for use. They all have a flow regulator, filter and a burette chamber (Fig. 3.13). In some cases, the chamber is graduated for precise measure-

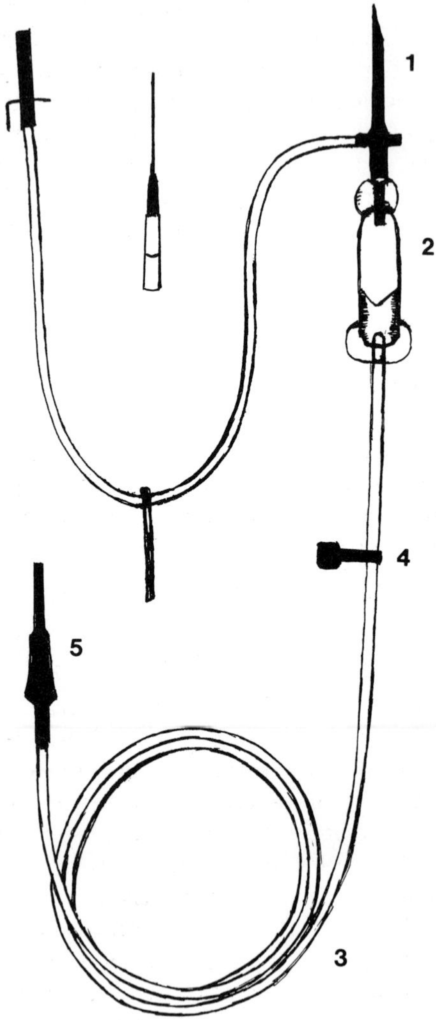

Fig. 3.13 Administration set for intravenous solutions (Baxter–Travenol). 1. Connectors with integral airways; 2. Drip-chamber with filter; 3. Tubing of 3 mm diameter; 4. Flow regulator; 5. Flashball injection site.

ment of dispensing fluid, particularly for use with children. Also there are 'Y' type sets to allow administration of two infusion fluids, alternately or simultaneously (Fig. 3.14). Some sets are solely for intravenous infusion of fluid, others for blood transfusion, and yet a third type for either blood or fluid infusion. Generally, the system used for blood transfusion has a filter with a relatively large pore size, and a so-called 'pump chamber' to permit changes from gravity flow to pressure administration. The pump is safe because it is a closed liquid system (with no air) operated by hand. The set for fluid infusion has a fine filter pore size and no pump chamber (Fig. 3.15). All sets have a flash ball injection site for supplementary medication.

Accessory equipment for intravenous feeding

Essential requirements for the delivery of nutrients into the blood stream are the intravenous catheters and infusion systems. In recent years, additional equipment has been designed to reduce the incidence of complications, or to facilitate administration and assist with nursing management (Fig. 3.16).

Flow control systems and pumps (Table 3.14)

The gravity 'self-running' infusion system has been used for a number of years without major problems. However, under certain circumstances, the gravity flow intravenous infusion systems do have some limitations. For instance, a system with only a manually controlled clamp to regulate the flow rate does require continual, or very frequent, observation so that solutions are administered at a constant rate and according to the prescribed time schedule. Rapid administration of hypertonic amino acid solutions not only decreases the amount utilized, but also results in unpleasant reactions in the patient. Irregularities in timing of administration may also result in an unexpected completion of the infusion with the risk of air embolism. However, the limitations of the gravity flow intravenous infusion systems do not prevent satisfactory administration of the infusion in the majority of patients requiring intravenous feeding in a general surgical/medical ward.

Apparatus concerned with flow rate and its control (Table 3.14) are flow controllers and pumps which control the drip rate or the volume.

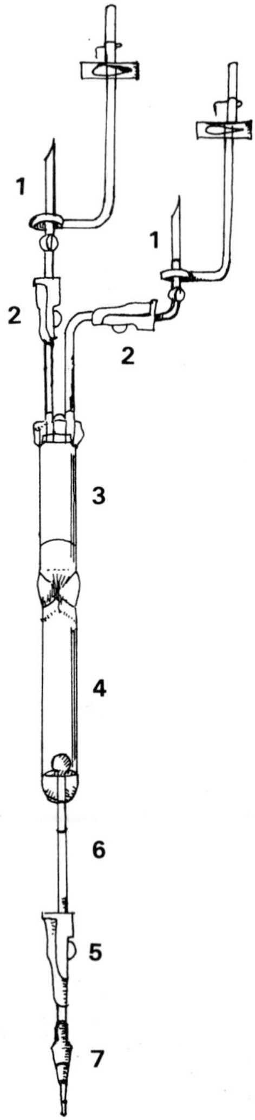

Fig. 3.14 Y-Type blood or solution administration set (Baxter–Travenol). 1. Connectors with integral airways; 2. Flow-regulator; 3. Drip-chamber with filter; 4. Hand-operated pressure pump for rapid administration if required; 5. Additional flow regulator; 6. 147 cm of 3 mm tubing; 7. Flashball injection site for supplemental medication.

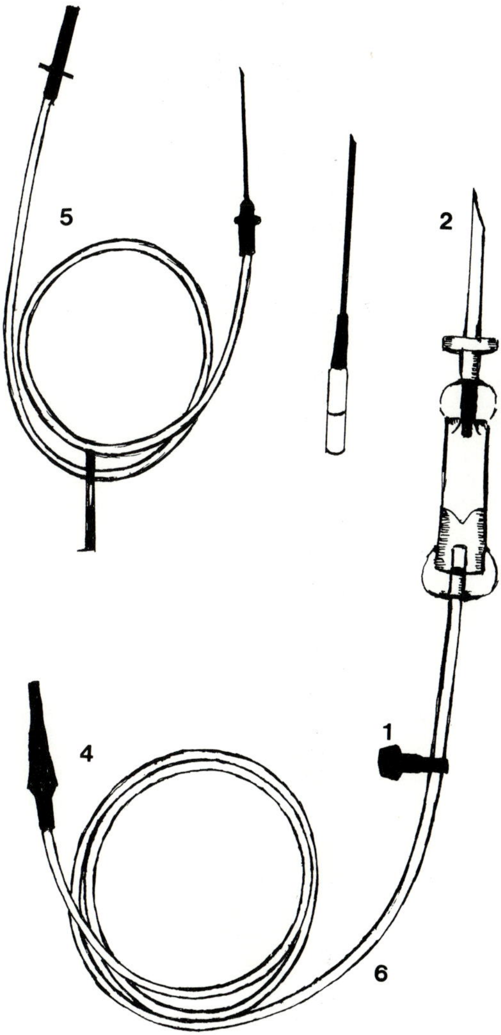

Fig. 3.15 Administration set for solution only (Baxter–Travenol). 1. Flow regulator; 2. Connector for solution container; 3. Drip-chamber with visible safety filter against inadvertant misuse for blood or blood derivatives; 4. Flashball injection site for supplemental medications; 5. Airway device; 6. Length of tubing 142 cm and 3 mm diameter. Note no pump chamber and visible filter.

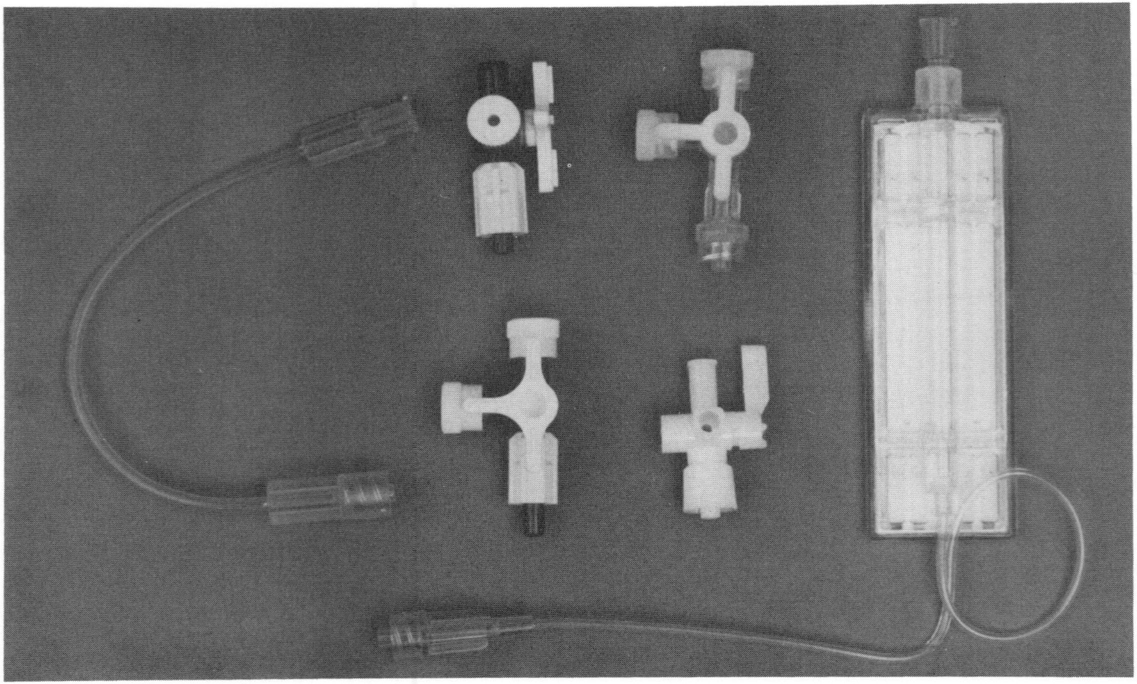

Fig. 3.16 *Accessory equipment for intravenous feeding (excluding flow regulators).* From left to right: *extension tube, 4 two-way taps, filter end line type. Note suitable taps are those with flat lower surface (taps in lower part of the figure) which lie comfortably on the skin.*

Table 3.14 Flow controller and pumps for intravenous feeding

Designation	*Manufacturer*	*Drip rate range*	*Battery/mains*	*Stand availability*
Gravity flow controller	Frenshore Ltd.	1–99 d.p.min	Mains	Yes
Gravity flow controller	Ivac UK	1–69 d.p.min	Mains or battery	Yes
Pump (linear peristaltic)	Imed Ltd.	1–99 d.p.min	Mains	Yes
Pump (linear peristaltic)	Ivac UK	1–99 d.p.min	Mains or battery	Yes
Pump (linear peristaltic)	Graseby Dynamics Ltd.	1–99 d.p.min	Mains	No
Pump (rotary peristaltic)	Vickers Ltd.	3–60 d.p.min (in 12 steps)	Mains	No

Flow controllers

These types of apparatus rely on gravity for the actual pressure of the flow, but automatically control the drip rate and therefore the flow. In a majority of these instruments a sensor is attached to the drip chamber to count the drops, and the rate is adjusted by operating the clamp acting on the delivery tube. An alarm system is also incorporated in the system to warn against increased resistance and under-infusion.

As the name implies, all drop-counter controllers operate by sensing the number of drops. The size of the drop does not affect the regulatory mechanism. Consequently, the total volume dispensed depends on the nature of the fluid and the administration set, which determines the volume of each drop. In short, the apparatus is a drop-counter and controller, not strictly a flow controller.

Ivac 231 and Frenshore IC_2 are examples of this type of controller.

Pumps

As the name implies, pumps exert pressure on the flow. If there is a blockage in the infusion system, the pressure may rise. If there is a displacement of cannula, a considerable extravasation may result.

There are two types of pumps available for intravenous infusion: the drip-rate and volumetric.

Drip-rate pumps combine the principle of a drip-counter with the application of pressure forcing the fluid through the administration set. A drop sensor is attached to the infusion set to control the rate of the drops which are then driven, by pressure, into the vein. The infusion rate is maintained in spite of the change in resistance. Therefore, in the presence of increased viscosity (related to the type of fluid), the flow rate is still maintained.

Volumetric pumps provide a constant flow in spite of change of drop size.

Filters and air 'bubble' eliminators

All solutions contain some particulate matter, and intravenous infusion solutions contain microbubbles of air, particles and, possibly, some micro-organisms in varying amounts and proportions. In recent years, in-line (added to the infusion system but not an integral part of the set) filters have been designed specifically to eliminate air bubbles by a vent system and retain particles and bacteria. It has been estimated that during extensive intravenous therapy a patient may receive up to 1000 million particles greater than 1 μm in size of paper, fibres, cotton, glass, flex and plastic material.

Any manipulations of the intravenous infusion can add many more particles to the final count. Infused particles have been related to granulomatous formation, pulmonary fibrosis and phlebitis. In the case of microbial infusion, it is clear that they are theoretically responsible for infective complications and septicaemia, bearing in mind the particular predisposition to the development of infection of some patients requiring intravenous therapy.

In-line filters for intravenous infusion are used extensively in the USA, and the National Coordinating Committee for Large Volume Parenterals (NCCLVP, 1979) has made some recommendations for their use. It is suggested that they are used in the following instances:

1. Patients receiving parenteral nutrition.
2. For the immune deficient or immune compromised individual receiving intravenous infusion.
3. Patients receiving infusions with many additives.

These recommendations have been the stimulus for the widespread use of in-line filters in the USA, but, in the UK, in-line filters are not extensively used for intravenous purposes, although microfilters are in common usage for blood transfusion. However, in future, more in-line filters may be used for intravenous feeding, and it is therefore of benefit to have some knowledge of their function and their limitations.

Ideally, the filter must be capable of retaining all particles and micro-organisms and prevent the entry of air bubbles into the vein, while not interfering with the flow rate. The filter should be of an 'end line' (i.e. attached near the catheter) type (synonymous with 'final' or 'add-on filter'). It must not alter or retain the chemicals or solutes from the intravenous solution, i.e. it can be used for all solutions. An ideal filter, possessing all these properties, is yet to be made. However, there are some currently available that possess most of them. Nevertheless, the available filters cannot presently be used when the intravenous feeding regime contains lipid, because the lipid emulsion blocks the filter. Nor can these filters be used for infusions of blood derivatives and substitutes.

Practical hints for the use of end-line filters in intravenous feeding are as follows:

1. It is important to have an idea of the pore size of the filter. If the filter is intended to retain micro-organisms, the membrane must have a pore size of less than 0.3 μm (one of the smallest organisms is *Pseudomonas diminuta* at about 0.3 μm).

2. An end-line type of filter, connected near to the catheter, should be used. Some filters are provided with a side-line downstream, allowing by-pass of the filter, if necessary, for injection of a drug incompatible with the infusion solution.

3. Lipid solutions must not be allowed to pass through the filter.

4. If the filter is required to remove air, then one provided with this capability should be used.

5. Blood micro-filters intended to remove micro-aggregates are not designed for filtration of intravenous feeding solutions. They are called 'micro-filters', but particles of even 100 μm can pass through, whereas the 'filters' for intravenous fluid infusion deal with particles of less than 1 μm. It is also worthwhile to point out that an administration set's filters (integral part of the set) have a pore size of over 150 μm. Table 3.15 shows some of the filters available in the UK.

Taps, extension tubes and connectors

An infusion system can be connected directly to the intravenous catheter, in which case there is no intervening connector, tap or extra tubing. In the majority of cases, however, it is necessary to have a two- or three-way tap in between the giving set and the intravenous catheter, and an extension tube, both of which facilitate nursing management.

The tap has several functions. It provides an alternate and/or a simultaneous infusion channel and aids in temporarily closing off the intravenous catheter, but keeping it *in situ* for re-usage, in which case the catheter is filled with heparinized saline solution and the tap closed to all outside positions. Finally, with certain provisos and precautions, it proves a channel for bolus administration of drugs when the infusion is not in progress, or is temporarily discontinued. The following points should be noted.

Table 3.15 Some of the filters available in UK

Designation	*Manufacturer*	*Type*	*Membrane rating (approximate pore size)*	*Special features*
Abbot IVEX-2	Millipor Corp.	End line (in line)	0.22 m	Side line No special air bubble removal
Pall FAE 020 LYL Ultipor	Pall Biochemical Ltd.	End line (in line)	0.20 m	Side line and air bubble removal
Braun Sterifix infusion filter	Gelman Corp.	End line	0.20 m	No side line No air bubble removal

The terminology for 'end line' filters varies. The terms 'final', 'final in line', 'end line' and 'add on' essentially mean the same thing, i.e. the filter is not part of the administration set, but is connected between the administration set and the catheter.

1. They must have a locking fitting (luer lock).
2. The open end of the tap must have a cap to protect the opening from any collection of debris or contaminated materials.
3. Experience shows that some taps do not sit well on the patients skin as they do not possess a flat surface.

Therefore, it is important to use taps designed for intravenous nutrition purposes.

Extension tubes with connectors are an accessory, but useful addition, for intravenous feeding infusion systems. They are multipurpose devices interposed between the catheter (or the tap) and the infusion set. Some provide a system of tubing for several simultaneous infusions (e.g. LS connectors by Braun). Others, such as the Vygon catheter extension tube with connectors (Fig. 3.17), provide an extension tubing which, when interposed between the catheter and the infusion set and because of its easy manipulation, facilitates nursing management. This may also reduce the risk of contamination.

These accessories are important for reducing any contamination of open and exposed 'ends'. A majority of the most recently developed devices are fitted with Luer or other locks.

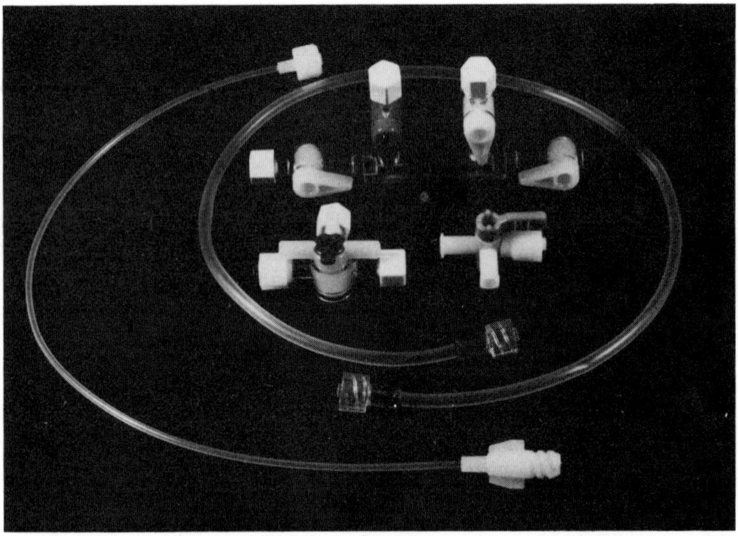

Fig. 3.17 Taps, extension tubes and connectors (Vygon).

14. Care of Infusion Systems

Once the intravenous infusion for parenteral nutrition is established, its care and survival remain the responsibility of the nursing staff. A majority of patients require intravenous infusion for several days and some may receive it for weeks, a few for even longer. It is important to realize the importance of intravenous feeding for a patient, and understand its potential dangers. Intravenous feeding constitutes the only channel of nutrition in patients with total parenteral nutrition and, therefore, the management of the intravenous infusion is vital. Much of the care of the patient with a central venous line for parenteral nutrition is concerned with minimizing the risk of complications (p. 146). Here, guidance is given in the technical management of the infusion.

PROVISION OF THE DAILY NUTRIENT AND FLUID REGIME

A daily intravenous regime is prescribed by a medical officer on an appropriate prescription chart, and should supply adequate nutrients and fluid for the needs of the patient.

In order to avoid confusion, and to ensure accuracy of the fluid balance measurement, it is invaluable to have a recording chart where both commencement and completion of the intravenous fluid container are recorded separately. The type of solution, volume and identity number of the container is recorded, and the time noted when it is commenced. On completion, or when taken down, the volume is recorded in a separate column and the time indicated. It is also helpful to chart at what time the infusion of the fluid in the container is due to be completed.

It is clearly important that a patient receives the prescribed nutrients and fluid within 24 hours and, therefore, it is necessary to ensure that the infusion is running at the correct rate. This task is made much less onerous if an infusion pump is used to regulate the rate of infusion. Otherwise frequent checking of the rate is needed.

It is also important to ensure that the fluid continues to run. If it stops for more than a very short period of time, the catheter may be blocked by a blood clot and the intravenous catheter need re-inserting. To minimize this risk, the next infusion unit must be checked to ensure it is ready to be put up without delay when required.

CHANGING THE NUTRIENT CONTAINER

Changing the nutrient container is essentially the same as changing any other intravenous container, but the potential hazards to a patient are greater. Therefore, a number of points are reiterated here.

1. The prescription and the nutrient container for infusion must be checked by two people, one of whom is normally a State Registered Nurse.
2. Because the nutrient solutions are an ideal media for bacterial growth, the container is carefully checked for cracks where organisms may have entered, and for any indications of deterioration, such as cloudiness of an amino acid solution. The expiry date is also checked.
3. Risk of infection is relatively high, and the possible consequences very serious. Therefore, every care must be taken to prevent any infection entering the infusion system. Thorough hand-washing before changing the bottle is essential, with particular attention to the dominant hand, between the fingers and backs of hands. These are the areas which researchers have found to be least well washed. Rings, of any sort, should not be worn as they result in a higher bacterial count on the hands. Even though sterile gloves are used before changing a nutrient container, this should not give a false sense of security because, having touched the infusion set, etc., they are no longer sterile.
4. Clearly, the top of the new container must be sterile to prevent bacteria being pushed through into the bottle. Care is always taken during removal from the old bottle and insertion into the new that the insertion point of the infusion set does not touch anything unsterile, otherwise the whole infusion set has to be changed.
5. In some units a face mask is worn when changing the nutrient container. The rationale for this is that, in exerting the force required to insert the thick infusion needle through the thick rubber bung of the bottle, it is difficult to avoid exhaling forcibly over the bottle and infusion needle—a mask at least diverts this flow of breath.

CARE OF THE INFUSION SYSTEM

The infusion system itself is discussed on p. 125, but there are certain principles in management which aim to maintain its functioning with the minimum of complications.

An intravenous feeding infusion system should not be used for the measurement of central venous pressure, blood transfusion, or the withdrawal of blood. All these result in blood flowing back into the catheter. If any are essential, then the catheter is rapidly flushed through with normal saline to ensure it is clear. Medications are never given through this system, as the risk of infection is increased.

As risk of infection increases with the length of time the administration set is used, the set must be changed every 24–48 hours and after blood transfusion. In practice, this is more likely to be undertaken regularly if the set, two- or three-way taps, extensions, etc., are all changed at approximately the same time every day.

Changing the infusion set

Figure 3.18 illustrates the equipment required. The procedure for changing the infusion system is planned to minimize the risk of two complications, i.e. risk of infection and air embolus, both of which are greater with a central venous line for parenteral nutrition than with an ordinary intravenous infusion.

It is essential that, in order to minimize the risk of disconnection of the infusion set from the catheter once the strapping, etc., has been removed, the patient is not left alone while the nurse goes to wash her hands. If at all possible, two nurses should undertake this procedure, an operator and assistant, but if this is impossible then sterile gloves must be worn to minimize risk of infection. A mask is always worn for this procedure and, in some units, a gown.

The following practice is recommended and, while it is neither original or necessarily the best, the method is practical and safe.

1. The new infusion set is filled slowly (to prevent air bubbles in the tubing) with the nutrient solution to be commenced. This procedure never utilizes a partly used nutrient infusion as this increases risk of infection. The protective device on the end of the tubing must be kept dry and remain in position until the set is needed.
2. A sterile two- or three-way tap is attached to a 2 ml syringe.

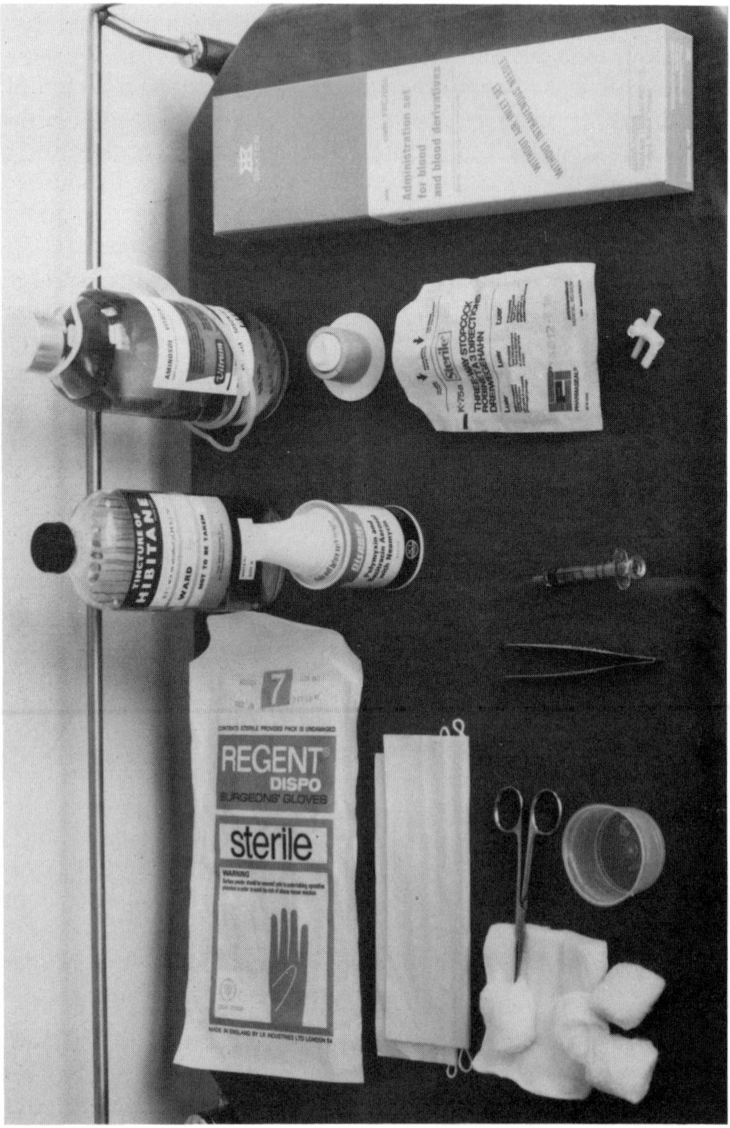

Fig. 3.18 Suggested equipment for changing the infusion set (see text).

3. The dressing and strapping over the catheter and tap are carefully removed.

4. The skin surrounding the catheter is cleansed, and the tap and point at which the set will be disconnected are cleaned with spirit.

5. The tap is turned off. The used administration set and tap are disconnected from the catheter and immediately replaced by a new tap attached to the syringe. At this point, the use of the Valsalva manoeuvre (the patient tries to breath out against closed mouth and pinched nose) will raise the intrathoracic pressure and prevent air being sucked into the catheter. Lying the patient flat also minimizes this risk as the venous pressure is then higher.

6. The tap is turned on and some blood aspirated into the syringe to check the patency of the catheter and remove any air which may have entered.

7. The tap is turned off, the syringe removed and the new administration set (already prepared) is attached.

8. The tap is turned on and the catheter flushed through with solution and the rate adjusted according to the schedule for administration. If working alone, one hand is used to adjust the rate (i.e. becomes 'unclean'), and the other hand remains 'clean' to apply the new dressing.

9. Polybactrin (or antibiotic spray or cream) is applied and covered by a dressing. A semi-permeable dressing, such as Op-Site, seals the entry of the catheter and allows observation of the insertion site.

10. The tubing near the two- or three-way tap must be securely fixed in position to ensure that the system cannot be pulled apart.

11. The rate of flow is adjusted as required.

DISCONTINUATION OF PARENTERAL NUTRITION

When parenteral nutrition is to be discontinued, the catheter is removed with similar precautions. The procedure is as follows:

1. After removal of the dressing and cleansing of the skin, any fixation stitch is removed.

2. The infusion is turned off and the catheter withdrawn firmly and smoothly, while pressure is applied with a gauze pad at the insertion site. Pressure is maintained for a short time. The catheter is placed on a sterile, waterproof towel or in a sterile container.

3. The skin is sprayed with Polybactrin (or other antibiotic spray) and a small dressing applied.

4. To check for the presence of infection, the tip of the catheter is cut off with sterile scissors or blade and sent for microbiological examination.

5. A chest x-ray is taken after catheter removal.

15. Monitoring Parenteral Nutrition Therapy

An important aspect of any treatment is the assessment of its efficiency in bringing about the expected and desired results. In this instance, assessment is made by monitoring a patient's progress and the safety of the nutritional therapy. At intervals, in the course of the treatment, a series of observations and specific tests are undertaken with the object of:

- assuring the safe progress of intravenous feeding and minimizing complications by early diagnosis and prompt treatment to prevent their full development;
- verifying the adequacy of the nutrients provided for the specific metabolic requirements of the patient, and checking the satisfactory maintenance of the nutritional state. Evaluating the benefit of the treatment.

These objectives are reached by using a number of relevant parameters measured at intervals in the course of intravenous therapy. The number and frequency of the parameters used depend on the type of patient under treatment, the available facilities and the objectives of the therapy. Thus, in a research situation, it may be desirable or even essential to measure many parameters at frequent intervals. However, in a purely clinical situation, both the number and the frequency of the tests applied are reduced to a realistic and minimum safe level for the conduct of treatment. However, without monitoring, intravenous feeding will not achieve its purpose, and complications may overshadow any potential benefits.

The monitoring of parenteral nutrition therapy is discussed under three headings: general monitoring of the patient; nutritional monitoring; and monitoring related to the technique.

General monitoring of the patient

Intravenous nutrition is of course only one aspect of a patient's treatment and care while in hospital. The condition and treatment being received will influence the observations carried out, but regular measurement of temperature, pulse and respiration are necessary. A rise in temperature is an important observation, as it may indicate the development of infection from the intravenous nutrition site.

A patient's general condition is naturally monitored during nursing care. The condition of the skin, hair, nails and the level of mobility and activity undertaken, as well as the patient's psychological state, all benefit as nutritional status improves. Any deterioration in the condition of the skin (pressure sore development) or wound (wound infection) is always noted and reported as nutritional needs may be increased.

Nutritional monitoring

In essence, nutritional monitoring relies on repetition of all or some of the tests used in the nutritional assessment of a patient (p. 52). In practice, some additional tests and observations are necessary; an inevitable consequence of this method of treatment.

Monitoring intake and fluid balance

The volume and type of administered nutrients must be clearly recorded and charted, so that it is possible to calculate the intake of energy, nitrogen and other nutrients. In addition, the volume of any other fluid intake and all sources of fluid loss (e.g. drainage, aspiration, wound discharge, as well as urine volume) are recorded to allow an accurate assessment of fluid balance. This is supplemented by regular weighing of the patient, as short-term alterations in weight are usually due to fluid changes. Obviously, weight should be recorded at the same time every day, and in approximately the same amount of clothing and, if possible, the same scales used, as scales can vary in accuracy.

Anthropometric measurements

In patients receiving parenteral nutrition, the triceps skin-fold thickness and mid-arm circumference (allowing calculation of mid-arm muscle circumference) is measured over 3 to 4 days (p. 56). In conjunction with bodyweight, this allows the monitoring of changes in body stores of nutrients.

Biochemical monitoring

Of the variety of possible laboratory tests which are employed to monitor various aspects of intravenous feeding, some are indispensable for the day-to-day conduct of the treatment, or are necessary for adjustment of the intravenous regime and are carried out daily. Other tests, important for assessment of the nutritional progress, are done less frequently. Yet, other tests are used with patients receiving prolonged total parenteral nutrition, or in research.

It must be emphasized, however, that the type and frequency of tests carried out depend on many factors, for instance, the type of patient (i.e. the condition from which the patient is suffering), the duration of total parenteral nutrition therapy and complications arising from intravenous feeding or related to the primary illness. Following extensive and complicated surgical operations, patients may require a few daily tests, others at frequent intervals. Those on artificial ventilation also require blood gas analysis and daily estimation of acid-base status, whereas in other patients this daily analysis may be totally unnecessary. Daily plasma electrolyte and urea estimations are monitored to correct promptly any aberrations which may be life-threatening. For instance, potassium depletion may bring about cardiac arrhythmias or arrest. Intravenous feeding with solutions of high glucose and amino acid content frequently produce hypokalaemia, requiring correction by the daily addition of potassium in the regime.

Blood sugar, serum and urine osmolality are advised by some to be carried out on an everyday basis, and in some cases these tests are indispensable. These daily measurements in a routine surgical or medical patient on intravenous feeding, with no hepatorenal insufficiency, is however questionable. Nevertheless, even in these patients, tests are carried out every 2 to 3 days, or more frequently if results prove to be abnormal. Blood gas analysis and acid-base status are particularly important in some patients with cardiorespiratory or renal problems, and the frequency of this test is determined by clinical judgement. Plasma albumin, protein, serum phosphate and urea are frequently measured in all cases. The biochemical profile is carried out by an Auto-Analyser, which estimates many of these biochemical parameters at the same time as the electrolytes. Thus, when a blood sample is dispatched to the laboratory for electrolyte and urea estimation, a number of other chemicals can be measured from the same sample.

Liver function tests are carried out at least every 3 to 4 days, or more often if indicated.

Other laboratory tests

In patients receiving long-term intravenous feeding, and/or with metabolic disorders, other tests are performed to prevent the development of nutritional deficiencies. These include the measurement of trace elements, particularly zinc and copper, essential fatty acids, plasma amino acid profile and plasma ammonia.

Urine

The urinary urea and electrolytes are measured, sodium being of particular importance. Abnormal constituents are determined and measured as required, dependent on the type of case and any abnormalities. In practice, urine is tested routinely each day on the ward. The tests for glucose and ketones are made twice daily.

Ward-testing of the specific gravity of urine is simple and informative and is also done daily. Ames Multistix-SG provides a close estimate of the specific gravity of urine by a test based on the ionic concentration of the urine.

Blood count

Full blood count, including haemoglobin, red and white blood cells, is carried out every 3 to 4 days.

Monitoring related to the technique

The infusion system (i.e. the giving set, catheter and accessory equipment concerned with the delivery of nutrients) should not be forgotten when monitoring the progress of parenteral nutrition. Many of the complications associated with the infusion system can be averted, or aborted, in the early stages. Regular change of the infusion set and accessories, such as connectors and taps, are discussed on p. 139. It is important to check the correct positioning of the catheter, integrity and hub, as well as secure fixation to the skin.

Clearly, the running of the intravenous infusion must be regularly monitored. When an electronic flow rate regulator or a pump is frequently used, observations are still needed to ensure their continued correct functioning.

16. Complications and their Prevention

As stated, intravenous feeding is an important therapeutic technique. However, in submitting a patient to this therapy, consideration must be given to the benefit which such treatment can offer and the risks involved in its application. The understanding and prevention of complications, which may lead to increased morbidity and mortality, greatly influence the success of treatment.

In intravenous feeding a number of diverse complications may occur, involving multiple factors. For the purposes of description, however, they are grouped as (1) complications of the infusion system and technique; (2) infective complications; and (3) metabolic complications.

COMPLICATIONS RELATED TO THE INTRAVENOUS INFUSION SYSTEM AND TECHNIQUE

Many complications of the intravenous infusion system are due to faulty techniques of catheter insertion and management.

Catheter displacement

Catheter displacement has different causes and consequences depending on whether a peripheral cannulation or a central venous catheterization is undertaken. Displacement of the cannula inserted into a peripheral vein usually creates phlebitis due to extravasation of nutrient solutions (often hyperosmolar) into the perivenous and subcutaneous tissues. In addition, such an event obviously interferes with the delivery of the nutrients to a patient. Occasionally the extravasation of the nutrient solution into the subcutaneous tissues will cause cellulitis and ulceration (Fig. 3.19). The incidence of this complication can be prevented by never using peripheral veins for parenteral nutrition. Beyond this, it can be detected early and the results minimized by regular monitoring of the intravenous infusion. The rate of infusion is checked frequently and a reduction in rate may indicate that fluid is running into the tissues. The site of cannulation is examined at least daily, or more frequently if necessary.

In the case of central venous catheterization, the malposition of the catheter may be for two different reasons:

1. The catheter may have been malpositioned from the start due to faulty technique by the operator. Such instances are more frequent when the percutaneous, infraclavicular route is used to place the catheter through the subclavian vein. Some of the commonly recorded examples of malpositioning of the catheter and the consequences are:

- Catheter tip in a vein other than the superior vena cava (Fig. 3.20).
- Catheter entering an artery such as the subclavian artery, with resulting haematoma and haemomediastinum.
- Catheter transpiercing the vein with extravasation of blood into the neck, the mediastinum, the pleural cavity or the pericardium causing haematoma in the neck, haemothorax or haemopericardium.
- Pneumothorax and surgical emphysema from the escape of air into the pleural space or the extrapleural tissue spaces.

2. The catheter may become displaced after it has been inserted. This complication is associated with accidental movements of the catheter during procedures, such as changing the dressing. During a change of dressing over the site of catheter insertion, the catheter may

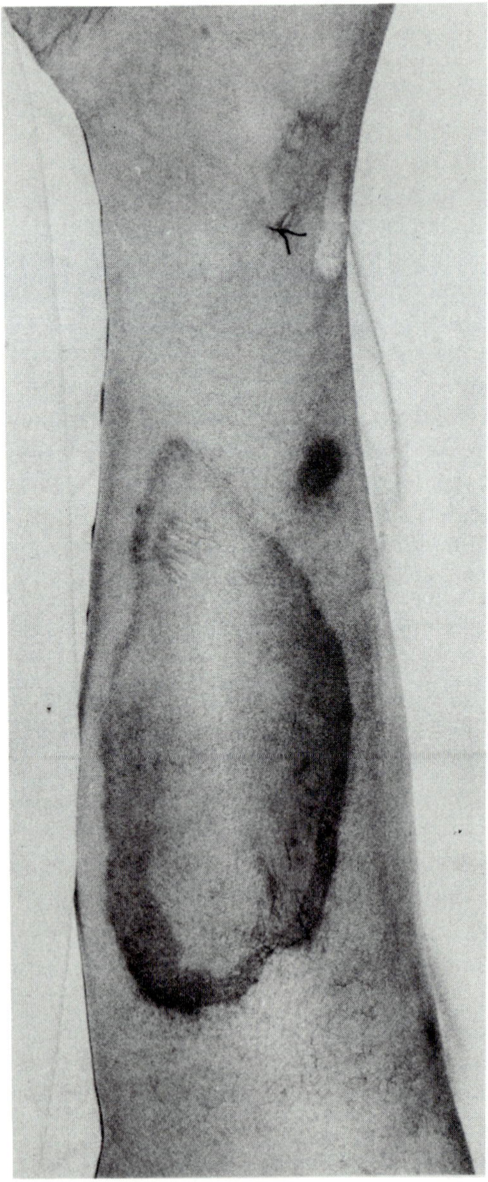

(b)

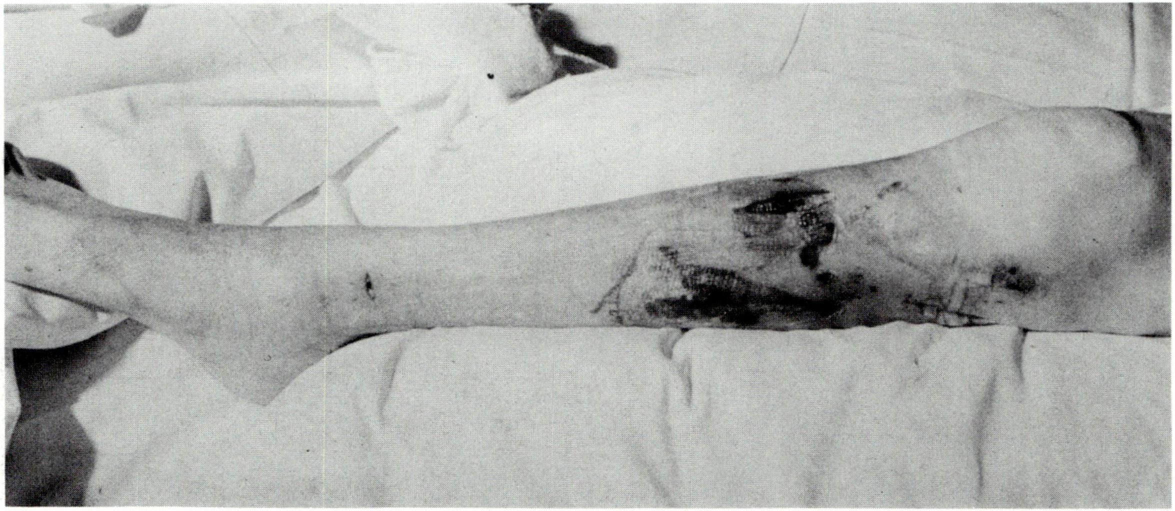

Fig. 3.19 (a) *The unacceptable face of parenteral feeding—cellulitis.* (b) *The unacceptable face of parenteral feeding—ulceration of the leg due to extra-vasation of nutrient solution.*

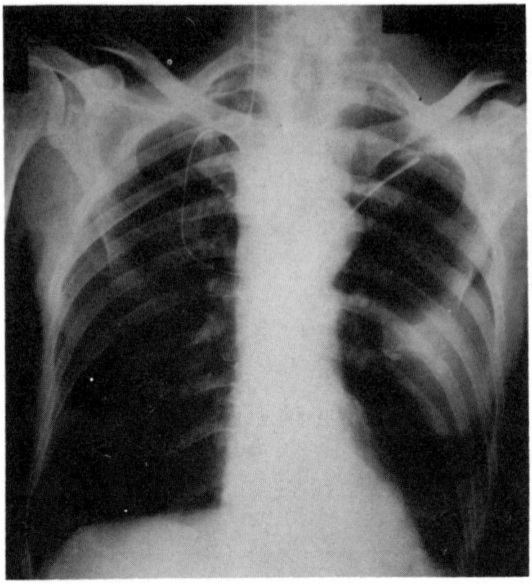

Fig. 3.20 Shows catheter inserted through the left subclavian vein, but entered into the right internal jugular vein moving towards the head.

adhere to the dressing and be partly withdrawn when it is removed, particularly if the percutaneous route is used. This is a particular risk when a semi-occlusive plastic adhesive dressing, such as Op-Site, is applied over the area of the venapuncture.

An intravenous catheter may also be displaced when it has not been securely fixed, and the patient's position is changed without specific attention to the intravenous infusion. Attention to detail in the initial insertion and fixing of the infusion catheter, and in the carrying out of dressings and moving the patient, will prevent these complications.

The consequences of catheter displacement are serious. In some cases the nutrient solution is delivered into the pleural space causing 'hydropneumothorax'. Not only does this complication cause respiratory and infective complications, but, in addition, it creates confusion about the state of nutritional intake which is obviously different from that delivered.

Any suspicion about the state of the catheter, or its position, affecting the flow of the intravenous infusion is checked and reported to a medical officer. The position of the catheter is then checked by x-ray and its replacement arranged if necessary.

Disturbance of flow of solution

Blocking of the catheter, or two-way tap or connector, obstructs the flow of solution. One of the commonest causes is interruption of the continuous flow of the infusion. The termination time of an infusion container must be foreseen so that the change is effected without delay and with the minimum of interruption to the infusion. The use of two infusion sets, connected to the catheter by a three-way tap, enables the immediate change over from one container to another to be completed without any disruption to the flow.

Air embolism

This can occur when a central venous catheter is opened to the air (e.g. during the change of the infusion set). The intrathoracic pressure is subatmospheric with respect to the external environmental pressure and, therefore, opening of the catheter to the air allows aspiration of air from outside into the catheter. The aspirated air enters the vein and moves into the heart. Air embolism can be fatal, or cause severe respiratory embarrassment. Air embolism is prevented by asking the patient to carry out the Valsalva manoeuvre (p. 141) or by putting him in the Trendelenburg position. By having the head lower than the body, the venous pressure is raised and air is not therefore aspirated into the vein.

Fracture of the catheter and catheter embolus

These complications are now extremely rare as they occurred in those systems where the catheter was inserted through the needle which then remained in position around the catheter. In these systems, any movement of the needle could damage the catheter and lead to a break, or even complete severance, of the catheter. The broken part of the catheter then entered the circulation as an embolus. These systems should not be used for parenteral feeding.

INFECTIVE COMPLICATIONS OF INTRAVENOUS FEEDING

Intravenous feeding involves insertion of the catheter and handling of equipment such as the giving set and two-way taps. It also involves procedures such as changing nutrient bottles, introduction of additives into the infusion solutions and change of dressing. All of these are potentially a source of contamination. In addition, two other factors are important in infective complications in intravenous feeding: (1) the particular susceptibility to infection of many of the patients receiving intravenous feeding; and (2) the possibility of self- or cross-infection which exists in some cases when, for instance, there is a co-existing wound or other infection.

It cannot be over-emphasized that in procedures related to the care of intravenous feeding, all involved in a patient's management must constantly bear in mind the danger of infection. The possible sources of infection in intravenous feeding are shown in Fig. 3.21. It can be seen that many factors involved in the infective complications can be dealt with in such a way as to minimize the risk.

Faulty technique in catheter placement by the operator may result in contamination and entry of micro-organisms into the body at the time of insertion. This is prevented by considering the procedure as a minor surgical operation, with a rigorous aseptic technique (p. 110). The use of an antiseptic and antibiotic spray over the site of the

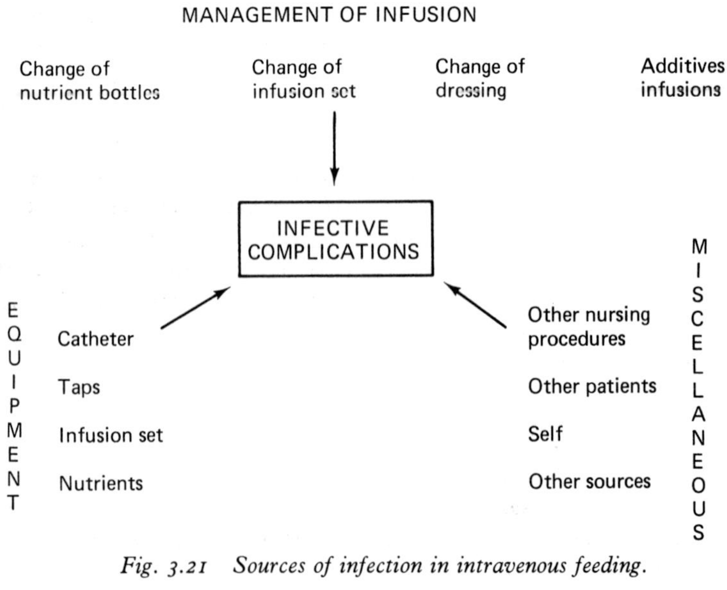

Fig. 3.21 Sources of infection in intravenous feeding.

insertion, forming a subcutaneous tunnel, and the use of a dressing such as Op-Site, all help reduce the risk of infection.

All manipulations of the feeding system, such as changing the nutrient bottle, are carried out aseptically to minimize risk of infection. The infusion system is changed every 24–48 hours because, after this time, the risk of infection rises. The dressing over the site of insertion is changed every 2–4 days. The use of a semi-occlusive, transparent dressing, such as Op-Site, appears to discourage bacterial growth and allow observation of the site. Considerable care must be taken to minimize any in-and-out movement of the catheter, as this can lead to bacteria being drawn back under the skin with the catheter.

Diagnosis and treatment of infective complications

Infective complications of intravenous feeding are local and/or general (septicaemia).

Local complications

Local infections occur at the site of the catheter insertion or on and around the veins. There may be simple local inflammation, cellulitis or pus formation. General signs of infection may be entirely in abeyance, but slight fever and leucocytosis may accompany these local signs.

When infection is local at the site of catheter insertion, wound swabs are taken and sent for culture. In patients with fever, with or without local infection, blood cultures are carried out and appropriate antibiotics prescribed. The intravenous catheter is removed and the tip sent to the microbiology laboratory for culture and sensitivity tests. If possible, the patient is not restarted on the infusion. In many patients, however, it is necessary to introduce, with vigorous antibiotic treatment, a new catheter at a different site.

General complications

Infection can be present as an acute episode of fever, malaise, tachycardia and rigor. A more gradual onset of all or some of the above symptoms may occur. In extreme cases there may be septicaemia with multiple abscesses in the lungs and other organs.

METABOLIC AND DEFICIENCY COMPLICATIONS

Metabolic acidosis

Many of the intravenous nutrients are acidotic, with a low pH. Some amino acid solutions contain a high concentration of chloride and, therefore, their administration causes excess retention of chloride and acidosis. Acidosis is corrected by administration of bicarbonate.

Uraemia

Some patients on parenteral nutrition develop increasingly high blood urea levels. In patients with intact renal function, this is associated with insufficient calorie intake in relation to nitrogen. Allowance of additional calories, particularly glucose, coupled with insulin, remedy this type of uraemia.

Hyperosmolality

The majority of intravenous nutrient solutions are hyperosmolar and their administration, particularly in large quantities, produces temporary hyperosmolality in some patients who are unable to adjust and accommodate the extra osmolar load. Serum hyperosmolality induces a series of neurological abnormalities culminating in hyperosmolar coma. This complication is prevented by monitoring the patient, particularly the urine glucose and the blood glucose content. Administration of insulin increases utilization of glucose and also remedies the hyperosmolality, which is caused by the high glucose content of the intravenous nutrient solution.

Hypophosphataemia

There are occasional reports of hypophosphataemia in patients receiving intravenous nutrition for long periods. This appears to be associated with large quantities of glucose intake in parenteral nutrition. Hypophosphataemia is reflected in a reduction in the red blood cells ATP content, and consequent fragility and haemolytic anaemia. Additional phosphate in the parenteral nutrition regimes will prevent this complication. It may also be necessary to administer additional phosphate when a large quantity of calories are derived from glucose.

Hypokalaemia

Infusion of glucose, particularly coupled with insulin, results in hypokalaemia. Administration of some amino acid solutions appears to have a similar effect. Because of the importance of the physiological action of potassium in the body, its frequent estimation in patients on parenteral therapy is essential. Hypokalaemia is corrected by appropriate additions to the intravenous infusion.

REFERENCES

Abbott W.E., Levy S., Krieger H. (1959). Metabolic change in surgical patients in relation to water, electrolytes, nitrogen and caloric intake. *Metabolism*; **8**: 847–861.

Copeland E.M., Dudrick S.J. (1978). The importance of parenteral nutrition as an adjunct to cancer treatment. International Symposium on Advances in Parenteral Nutrition, Bermuda 1977 Proceedings, pp. 473–499. Lancaster: M.T.P. Press.

Cuthbertson D.P. (1930). The disturbance of metabolism produced by bony and non-bony injury with notes on certain abnormal conditions of bones. *Biochem. J.*; **24**: 1244–1263.

Dudrick S.J., Wilmore D.W., Vars H.M., Rhoads J.E. (1969). Can intravenous feeding as a sole means of nutrition, support growth in the child and restore weight loss in an adult? An affirmative answer. *Ann. Surg.*; **169**: 974–984.

Fomon S.J. (1967). *Infant Nutrition*. Philadelphia: W.B. Saunders.

Grotte G. (1971). Nutrition parentérale du nourrisson. In *Solutés de Substitution Rééquilibration Metabolique* (Nahas, Viars, eds.), pp. 509–515. Paris: Librairie Arnette.

Grotte G., Jacobson S., Wretland A. (1976). Lipid and peripheral technique in parenteral nutrition. In *Total Parenteral Nutrition* (Fischer J.E., ed.), pp. 335–362, Boston: Little Brown and Co.

Jacobson S., Webster P.O. (1977). Balance study of twenty trace elements during total parenteral nutrition in man. *Brit. J. Nutrition*; **37**: 107–126.

Johnston I.D.A., Marino J.D., Stevens J.Z. (1966). The effect of intravenous feeding on the balance of nitrogen, sodium and potassium after operation. *Brit. J. Surg.*; **53**: 855–889.

Johnston I.D.A., Tweedle D.E.F., Spivy J. (1972). Intravenous feeding after surgical operation. In *Parenteral Nutrition* (Wilkinson A.W., ed.), p. 189. Edinburgh: Churchill Livingstone.

Lee H.A. (1974). *Parenteral Nutrition in Acute Metabolic Illness.* New York: Academic Press.

Moghissi K., Teasdale P.R. (1980). Parenteral feeding in patients with carcinoma of the oesophagus treated by surgery; energy and nitrogen requirements. *J. Parent. Ent. Nutr.*; **4**: 371–375.

Moore F.D. (1959). *Metabolic Care of the Surgical Patient.* Philadelphia: W.B. Saunders.

N.C.C.L.V.P. (1979). Recommendation for Action on an Important Problem Regarding Large Volume Parenterals: Problems and Benefits of In-line Filtration. 30th Nov.

Passmore, R. (1969). Body size and composition. In 'Recommended Intakes of Nutrients for the United Kingdom'. Reports on Public Health and Medical Subjects, No. 120 (D.H.S.S.). London: H.M.S.O.

Peaston M.J.T. (1966). Design of an intravenous diet of amino-acids and fat suitable for intensive patient care. *Brit. Med. J.*; **2**: 388–390.

Recommended Dietary Allowances, 7th Ed. (1968). Washington: Natn. Academ. of Sciences.

Ricour C., Millot M., Balsan S. (1975). Phosphorus depletion in children on long term total parenteral nutrition. *Acta Paediat. Scand.*; **64**: 385–392.

Scribner B.H., Cole J.J., Christopher T.G. *et al.* (1970). Long term total parenteral nutrition. The concept of an artificial gut. *J. Amer. Med. Ass.*; **212**: 457–463.

Shils M.E. (1972). Minerals in total parenteral nutrition. In A.M.A. Symp. *Total Parenteral Nutrition*, pp. 92–114.

Stell P.M. (1970). Esophageal replacement by transposed stomach. *Archs. Otolar.*; **91**: 166–170.

Tweedle D.E.F., Johnston I.D.A. (1971). Factors affecting the metabolic expenditure of surgical patients. *Brit. J. Surg.*; **58**: 771–774.

Van Larsen V., Brockner J. (1965). Nitrogen balance and operative stress. *Acta. Chir. Scan.*; *Suppl.*; **343**: 191.

Wilmore D.W., Groff D.B., Bishop H.C., Dudrick S.J. (1969). Total parenteral nutrition in infants with catastrophic gastro-intestinal anomalies. *J. Paediat. Surg.*; **4**: 181–189.

Wretlind A. (1972). Complete intravenous nutrition. Theoretical and experimental background. *Nutr. Metabol. Suppl.*; **14**: 1–57.

FURTHER READING

Benotti P.N., Bothe A., Miller J.D.B., Bistrian B.R., Blackburn G.L. (1976). Cyclic hyperalimentation. *Compr. Ther.*; **2**: 27–36.

Dudrick S.J., MacFadyen B.V., Van Buren C.T., Ruberg R.L., Maynard A.T. (1972). Parenteral hyperalimentation, metabolic problems and solutions. *Ann. Surg.*; **176**: 259–264.

Fischer J.E., ed. (1976). *Total Parenteral Nutrition.* Boston: Little Brown and Co.

Fischer J.E. (1979). Hyperalimentation. *Med. Clin. N. Amer.*; **63**(5): 973–983.

Heird W.C., Dell R.B., Driscoll J.M., Grebin B., Winters R.W. (1972).

Metabolic acidosis resulting from intravenous alimentation mixtures containing synthetic amino-acids. *N. Eng. J. Med.*; **287**: 943–948.

Hill G.H., ed. (1981). *Nutrition and the Surgical Patient*. Edinburgh: Churchill Livingstone.

Johnston I.D.A., ed. (1978). *Advances in Parenteral Nutrition*. Lancaster: M.T.P. Press.

Lee H.A. (1974). *Parenteral Nutrition in Acute Metabolic Illness*. London: Academic Press.

Michigan Nurses Association, Curn Project (1981). *Using Research to Improve Nursing Practice : Intravenous Cannula Change*. New York: Grune and Stratton.

Moghissi K. (1979). A technique of superior vena caval catheterisation for prolonged intravenous feeding. *J. Roy. Coll. Surg. Edinburgh*; **24**: 178–179.

Phillips I., Meers P.D., D'Arcy P.F., eds. (1976). *Microbiological Hazards of Infusion Therapy*. Lancaster: M.T.P. Press.

Riella M.C., Broviac J.W., Wells M., Scribner B.H. (1975). Essential fatty acid deficiency in human adults during total parenteral nutrition. *Ann. Intern. Med.*; **83**: 786–789.

Shenkin, A., Wretlind A. (1978). Parenteral nutrition. *World Rev. Nutr. Dietetics*; **28**: 1–111.

Silk D.B.A., Lieberman D.P., Sharrot P. (1978). Parenteral nutrition. *Hosp. Update*; **4**(10): 611–621.

SECTION IV

Enteral Nutrition

Enteral nutrition is a more 'normal' type of feeding in that it is using the gastrointestinal tract for the digestion and absorption of nutrients. However, to ensure safe practice and adequate feeding, both knowledge and skill are required. This mode of feeding is largely the province of the nurse and her abilities determine the success of this therapeutic tool.

The same plan, as outlined in Section III, is proposed.

17. Introduction

Enteral feeding is artificial nutrition via the alimentary tract. In the nutritional field, enteral feeding is the supply of blenderized made-up food, commercially available nutrients or an elemental diet, which are taken by mouth or delivered into the gastrointestinal tract through nasogastric, oesophagostomy, gastrostomy or jejunostomy tubes. Since nutrition via the alimentary tract is the physiological way of receiving nutrients, enteral rather than intravenous feeding offers a simple method of artificial feeding. In fact the relative simplicity of enteral, compared with parenteral, feeding is responsible for its recent popularity and widespread interest in clinical use. It must, however, be emphasized that there is no competition between the two methods of artificial feeding and, in many instances, there is a need for both methods to be employed at different times during illness. As found by Jones (1975), the apparent simplicity of enteral feeding may mean that its management is left to junior nurses with inadequate experience and knowledge. It is therefore essential that care is taken in the detail of administration of the feeding programme.

Enteral feeding is relatively simple because the route of delivery of nutrients is through the natural 'feeding system', i.e. the alimentary tract. However, the delivery of nutrients by this route does not equate with normal nutrition. Enteral feeding is still an artificial system of nutrition and is regarded as a therapeutic method requiring attention in its detail.

When enteral feeding is considered as a 'therapeutic method', it becomes clear that its effectiveness is dependent on the adequacy of the regime and the efficiency of its administration.

While parenteral feeding requires considerable nursing involvement, enteral feeding is even more the responsibility of nursing staff.

INDICATIONS AND SELECTION OF PATIENTS

Theoretically, enteral feeding may be employed in all patients requiring artificial nutrition providing that:

1. The alimentary tract is anatomically intact and physiologically functional with normal absorptive capabilities.

2. The nutrients are easily introduced and accommodated in the alimentary tract.
3. Nutrient solutions of suitable composition and consistency are available for the enteral method of feeding.

These conditions may not of course be fulfilled in all patients. However, in the vast majority of medical (and many of the surgical) patients requiring nutritional support, the alimentary tract is functional and enteral feeding can be used. Enteral feeding can be used either as a supplementary or total nutritional support.

Enteral feeding for supplementary nutritional support

At present, malnutrition is not the primary reason for most hospital admissions, but a closer look at patients in a hospital ward will indicate a high incidence of malnutrition. This is particularly so among the elderly (many of whom are not acutely ill), and undernourishment has a direct relevance to their hospitalization. This is further substantiated by the fact that, in some cases, malnutrition is so severe as to require urgent nutritional therapeutic measures. In addition, undernourishment (relative starvation) superimposed on any illness increases the severity of the latter, and reduces the chance of recovery. These facts suggest that artificial nutritional support is required, not only in severely or moderately malnourished patients, but also in those on the borderline of being nutritionally deficient and who may become severely malnourished if not supported. In many patients in this group, the malnutrition is an 'incidental' finding and, as the easiest method of nutritional support is by the enteral route, the commonest candidate for supplementary enteral feeding is the malnourished patient in hospital. There are also those who have neglected their nutrition, or, whilst in hospital for 'an illness', have received treatment for their illness but have been nutritionally neglected.

Indications for total enteral feeding

Apart from the above group of 'incidental' patients, there are others who require nutritional therapy not only as a supplementary support, but as the method of providing their total daily nutritional requirements. In many of these patients, malnutrition is caused directly by disease, e.g. patients with granulomatous disease of the gastrointestinal tract or short bowel syndrome. Theoretically there are only a few instances where enteral feeding cannot be used, e.g. major surgery of the upper alimentary system, or a non-functional gastrointestinal tract. Bearing this in mind, enteral feeding is successfully used in the following conditions:

- Pre-operative preparation of patients.
- Obstructive oesophageal lesions.
- Gastrointestinal fistula.
- Short bowel syndrome.
- Granulomatous disease of gastrointestinal tract.
- In burns.
- Adjunct to cancer chemotherapy.

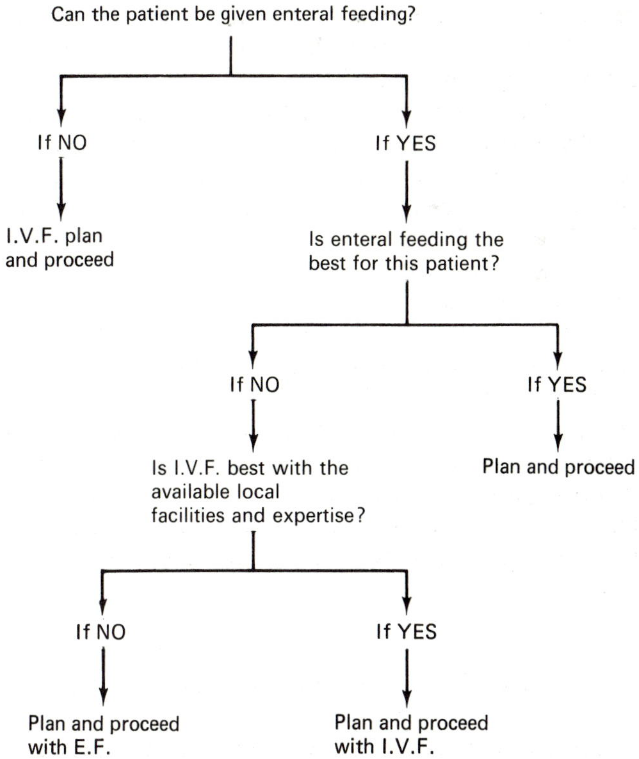

Fig. 4.1. Enteral feeding.

In some of these conditions, enteral feeding may not be the method of choice, but its relative simplicity may influence the clinician towards it.

In acute metabolic conditions, parenteral feeding may be employed first and then followed by the enteral method for maintenance of the therapy.

In practice, once the need for nutritional support is recognized, the question should be asked: Can the patient be given enteral feeding (*see* Fig. 4.1)?

18. Nutritional Requirements and Selection of Nutrients

Nutritional requirements for enteral feeding do not differ from that for intravenous feeding and either should supply a complete diet containing adequate and balanced quantities of water, energy, nitrogen (proteins), minerals and vitamins.

The quantitative data of nutritional requirements of the body in health is discussed on p. 32. In illness, basic requirements are increased to the level which covers the extra needs of metabolism due to the disease (p. 93).

In practice, the planning of the daily regime comprises of the following steps:

1. Assessment of the basic daily nutritional (including water) requirements for age, sex and bodyweight.
2. Adjustment and upgrading of the nutrient allocation for the extra requirements due to increased metabolism per kg of bodyweight.
3. Calculation of total daily water, energy, protein and other requirements for the patient under consideration related to his weight.
4. Selection of nutrient solutions and volume which best fulfil the calculated requirements.

If any additional energy or minerals are needed then the appropriate adjustments are made.

SELECTION OF NUTRIENT SOLUTIONS

Some of the commercially available nutrient solutions for enteral tube feeding are shown in Table 4.1. However, solutions containing the complete nutritional requirements of the diet still fall short of an ideal feed for enteral nutrition. At least two additional properties are required, namely a pleasant taste and tolerability by the body. None of these nutrient solutions can be said to have a pleasing taste. The inclusion of flavouring additives have not, on the whole, succeeded in making the solutions particularly pleasant, although they have made some more tolerable. When discussing the taste of solutions used for enteral feeding, two factors are relevant. First, many patients requiring artificial nutrition also have an alteration of taste and olfactory perception as a result of their illness. For instance, loss or alteration of taste is commonly observed in patients with extensive neoplasia. Second, in some cases, the after-taste of the preparation (that is following ingestion or administration) can be more displeasing than the actual taste when taking the nutrients.

In considering tolerability unrelated to taste, the osmolarity of the nutrient solution is an important consideration. A hyperosmolar liquid solution introduced into the alimentary tract can act in the same way as an osmotic laxative in producing a bowel action, and can cause diarrhoea.

At present, the general consensus of opinion is that there is no advantage in using an elemental diet instead of solutions containing a 'complete diet' in bottles or cans. There is also no advantage in a 'kitchen-prepared solution' over the commercially prepared ones. With the dietician's involvement, however, there is a definite indication for the hospital catering department to prepare appropriate feeds, using milk and such preparations as *Build-up* or *Complan*, for supplementation by mouth. With enteral tube feeding, using commercial preparations, it is advisable to take note of the following:

1. Most nutrient solutions for enteral feeding are hypertonic, and their bolus introduction causes gastrointestinal symptoms (diarrhoea, distension) therefore:

- they are given by continuous drip and not bolus;
- they are diluted, at least at the start of enteral feeding;
- at the beginning of feeding, half, or even a quarter, strength solution is used, gradually building up to a full concentration in 4–5 days.

Table 4.1 Nutrient solutions for enteral feeding

Brand name	*Manufacturer*	*Presentation*	*Volume*	*Total energy*	*Total nitrogen*	*Osmolality mosmol/kg*	*Vitamins*	*Minerals*	*Gluten*	*Lactose*
Ensure	Abbot	Bottle	235 ml	240 kcal	1.4 g	380	+	+	–	–
		Tin	235 ml	240 kcal	1.4 g	380	+	+	–	–
Ensure Plus	Abbot	Tin	235 ml	340 kcal	2.1 g	460	+	+	–	–
Build-up	Carnation	4 sachets per box	150 g	124 kcal/sachet	1.3 g		+	+	–	–
Triosorbon	E. Merck	Sachet	85 g	400 kcal	2.5 g	238	+	+	–	–
Complan	Farley	Packet (powder)	450 g	1000 kcal/pkt	7.2 g/pkt		+	+	–	–
Nutrauxil	KabiVitrum	Bottle	500 ml	500 kcal	3.0 g	350	+	+	–	–
Isocal	Mead and Johnson	Can	355 ml	375 kcal	1.9 g		+	+	–	–
Clinifeed 400	Roussel	Tin	375 ml	400 kcal	2.4 g	450	+	+	–	+
Clinifeed 500	Roussel	Tin	375 ml	500 kcal	4.8 g	810	+	+	–	+
Clinifeed LLS	Roussel	Tin	375 ml	500 kcal	3·6 g	665	+	+	–	–
Caloreen	Roussel	Resealable pack	5 kg	4 kcal/g		24.1% = 130	–	–	–	–
Vivonex Standard	Eaton Labs.	Sachet	80 g	290 kcal/sachet	0.98 g/sachet		+	+	–	–
Vivonex HN	Eaton Labs.	Sachet	80 g	300 kcal/sachet	2.00 g/sachet		+	+	–	–

Iso-osmolar nutrient solutions are used with theoretical advantage. However, if used over long periods of time, it is important to ensure that the intake of nutrients is adequate.

19. Routes and Techniques of Enteral Feeding

There are many ways of providing nutrients via the alimentary tract, but supplementary oral feeding and tube feeding are the most commonly used.

SUPPLEMENTARY ORAL FEEDING

When there is no obstructive lesion of the alimentary tract, and when the tract is anatomically and functionally intact, this method may be used to provide a high calorie and protein diet. Such a diet is planned by the nutritional team according to the needs of the patient. The dietician and the catering staff are consulted to provide a suitable and tasty regime, which is prepared in the hospital kitchen. Alternatively a manufactured nutrient mixture may be used as supplementary to that eaten by the patient, in which case the matter of taste is an important consideration in selecting the brand. None of the currently commercially available products for enteral feeding can be said to be tasty, but some can be flavoured and are tolerable. They are often more palatable to patients when cold, although some patients may be more able to tolerate them at room temperature.

When the enteral feeding is only supplementary, as can be the case in many instances, sip-feeding may be used. That is, patients are given the nutrient solution half-an-hour to one hourly and encouraged to sip and finish it before the next feed is due. Accurate recording of the amount actually taken (not the amount given to the patient) is essential. The supplementary feeds must be given at fairly frequent intervals (in small quantities if necessary) so that they are taken when cold from the refrigerator.

TUBE FEEDING

The principle of tube feeding is to bypass the mouth and to introduce the liquid (or liquidized nutrient solution) into the stomach or jejunum (Fig. 4.2). The follow methods are in common use.

Nasogastric tube feeding

This is the commonest form of enteral feeding used in hospitals. It is based on the introduction of a catheter through the nostril, passing through the nose, pharynx and the oesophagus into the stomach. The liquid food is then delivered directly into the stomach through the

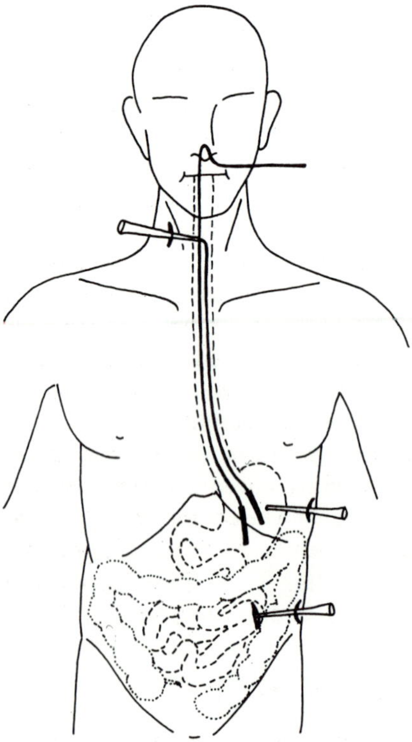

Fig. 4.2 Routes of enteral feeding (from above downwards): 1. Nasogastric tube; 2. Oesophagostomy; 3. Gastrostomy; 4. Jejunostomy.

tube. It is important to ensure that the nutrients are actually delivered into the stomach, and not totally or partially in the oesophagus (or trachea!).

The standard nasogastric tubes (Ryle's tubes) used for decompression of the gastrointestinal tract are wide-bore, and generally unsuitable for enteral feeding purposes. Not only are they uncomfortable for long periods, but are likely to cause gastro-oesophageal reflux oesophagitis, followed later on by oesophageal stricture formation (p. 185).

Preparation for passing a nasogastric tube

Before passing a nasogastric tube, it is necessary to prepare the patient psychologically, as the success of nasogastric tube feeding depends not only on the planning and the delivery of the nutrient by the nutritional team, but to a great extent on the understanding and the cooperation of the patient. It has been demonstrated in a number of research studies by Johnson (1976) that giving information about the sensations to be experienced, as well as the procedure to be carried out, helps the patient to be less anxious. Therefore, an explanation of what is going to be done, why, and how it will feel helps to mentally prepare the patient to cope better when they feel the tube being passed through their nostril and down the back of the throat, which can be uncomfortable, but does not hurt. However, the tube passing at the back of the throat may make them gag and feel that they want to vomit, but if they continue to breath steadily, and swallow when asked, the tube will be able to pass quickly and easily.

Some patients are extremely nervous of having 'anything passed' in their throat and have to be carefully managed. A sedative prior to passing the tube will help alleviate this situation.

Patients with infected teeth and nasopharynx are given mouth washes. In old and debilitated patients, the nose, mouth and nasopharynx is cleaned and sucked clear of purulent secretions. Once the preparation is satisfactorily completed, the equipment is brought to the patient on a tray, or preferably on a trolley (p. 170).

Techniques for placing the tube

According to the circumstances, and the type of facilities available, either of the following three techniques may be used for placing the tube.

1. Placement in the ward.
2. Placement under radiological control in the intensive care unit, x-ray department or the operating theatre, when an x-ray image intensifier is available.
3. Endoscopic placement. This method is particularly recommended when patients have to undergo endoscopic examination of the alimentary tract.

Except for cases where the placement is endoscopically undertaken, the patient is prepared, as described above, and helped into an upright position, if possible. Figure 4.3 shows the equipment required, which is as follows:

- Nasogastric tube.
- Lubricant (such as K.Y. Jelly) and swabs.
- 20 ml syringe and bowl.

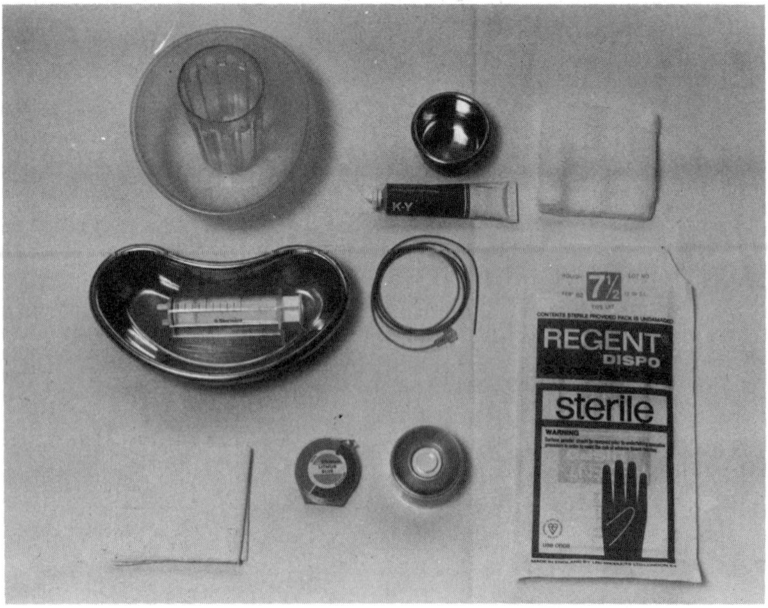

Fig. 4.3 Suggested equipment for insertion of nasogastric tube (enteral feeding). From left to right—Top row: *Bowl with drinking glass, gallipot, swab.* Middle Row: *Kidney dish with 20 ml syringe, fine bore nasogastric tube, KY jelly lubricant.* Bottom row: *Towel (to protect patient's clothing), litmus paper, adhesive tape, sterile gloves.*

- Litmus paper (for testing).
- Glass of water.
- Adhesive tape (for fixing the tube to nose).
- Gloves to protect the nurse and, more importantly, the weak patient from the risk of infection.

The procedure is carried out as follows. If the tube has a wire introducer, this is introduced into the tube—well-lubricated to permit easy withdrawal. The tube itself (with its introducer in place) is also lubricated. The tube is then passed gently through the nostrils. The passage of the tube through the pharynx provokes nausea and a sensation of vomiting, but this is usually averted by reassurance and allowing the patient to swallow saliva or drink some water. The patient should not breath very deeply at this stage (as usually is the practice for nauseated patients), particularly if a fine bore catheter is used in a patient with an obstructive oesophageal lesion or diminished swallowing reflex, as this may encourage the tube to enter the trachea. The tube is gently advanced for at least 50 cm. The introducer is then withdrawn and the correct position of the tube in the stomach checked. This can be done in one or more of the following ways.

1. Auscultatory method. Injection of air into the tube produces a bubbling noise which can be heard by concomittent auscultation of the epigastric region when the tube is in the stomach.
2. Radiological check. An antero-posterior x-ray view of the lower chest and upper abdomen shows the position of the tube and its tip (which is radio-opaque) in the stomach (Fig. 4.4).
3. Injection of a few drops of sterile water into the tube provokes coughing if the tube is accidentally introduced into the trachea.
4. When the tube has a medium (and not very fine) bore, its external (nostril) end is introduced under water and the epigastric area gently pressed. When the tube is in the stomach bubbles of air will be shown.
5. Suction of the tube in some cases may be useful, particularly when the tube is not of the very fine bore variety. The aspirated fluid is tested for acid gastric juices with litmus paper.

Once the position of the tube is checked, it is fixed to the nose and then to the forehead or the cheek. The latter tends to be more comfortable, is out of the visual field, and does not interfere with the wearing of spectacles. If the nose is sprayed (protecting the eyes) with tincture of benzoin, then sleek (waterproof strapping) used to fix the tube to the nose sticks well, even if the patient is sweating, and soreness rarely results (Fig. 4.5).

When the tube is positioned correctly, the end (male luer lock) connector is joined to the administration system which, in turn, is attached to the nutrient reservoir. The system is filled, free of air locks, before being connected to the nasogastric tube.

Gastrostomy and jejunostomy enteral feeding

In certain conditions, nasogastric tube feeding is not possible, (e.g. in

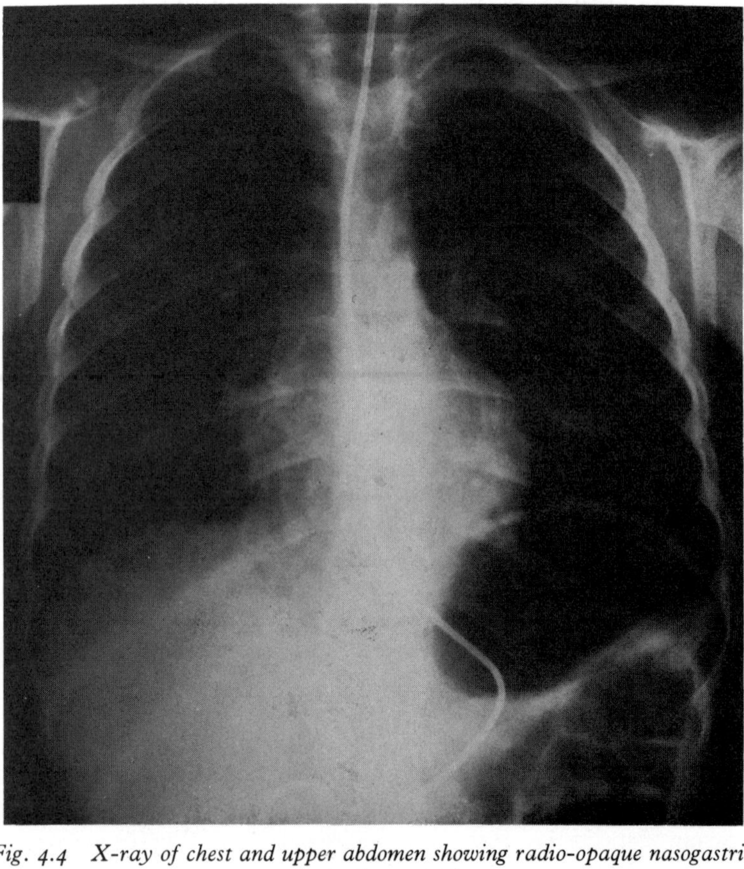

Fig. 4.4 X-ray of chest and upper abdomen showing radio-opaque nasogastric tube in the stomach.

total obstruction of the oesophagus), or it may be advantageous to introduce the nutrient directly into the stomach or jejunum, e.g. in cases of accidental rupture of the upper oesophagus. In these circumstances, a gastrostomy or jejunostomy is established (Fig. 4.2). Placing a gastrostomy or jejunostomy tube is an operative procedure

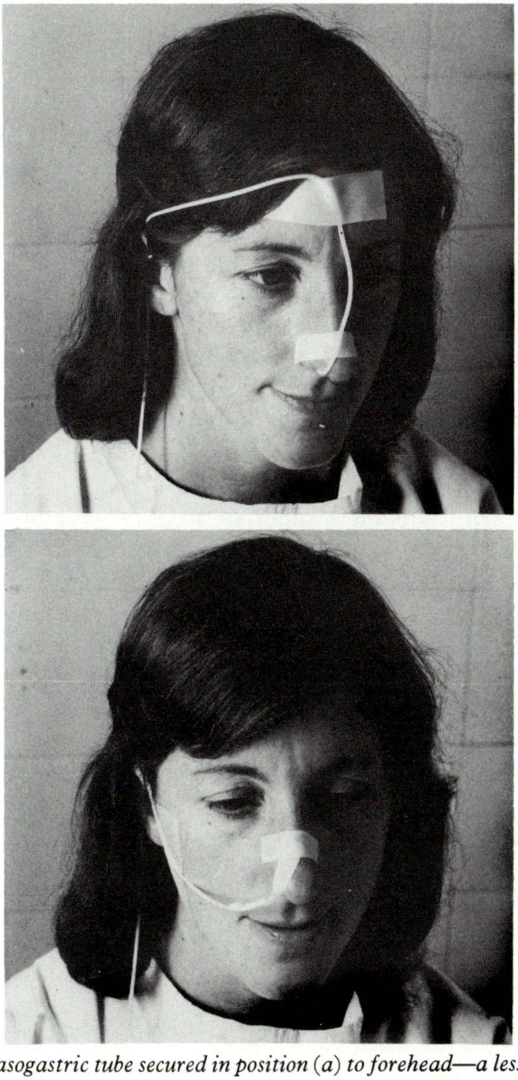

(*a*)

(*b*)

Fig. 4.5 *Nasogastric tube secured in position (a) to forehead—a less satisfactory method than (b) attached to cheek and passed over the ear.*

carried out in the operating theatre, usually under general anaesthesia.

Preparation for feeding gastrostomy

It is important to explain simply, but clearly, to the patient the reasons for the operation. It is also essential to communicate with the patient's relatives. Establishing these forms of enteral feeding requires an operation, and this can create fears and anxiety in the patient's mind (and the relatives). It has been shown by many researcher (Hayward, 1975) that giving patients accurate information about the pre-operative preparation (fasting, giving of premedication, being anaesthetized) and postoperative circumstances (where they will wake up, presence of drains, etc.) helps to minimize anxiety. The skin is prepared as for any surgical operation.

The surgeon performing the feeding gastrostomy or jejunostomy usually participates in the planning of the patient's nutrition, and chooses an appropriate tube.

On return of the patient to the ward, routine postoperative observations are carried out until a stable condition is maintained. For a few hours there may be reduced bowel activity and therefore a gastrostomy, in particular, may need hourly aspiration. Clearly, feeding cannot begin immediately.

At the start of feeding it is important to begin with diluted isotonic feeds, and aspirate at intervals to prevent distension of the stomach and reflux of gastric contents back to the oesophagus. This happens if the patient is weak and the stomach over-distended with fluid, particularly when the patient is in a recumbent position.

After a few days, there is often some leak of gastric juice around the gastrostomy tube. A protective paste (e.g. Aluminium paste, Karaya gum) should be used on the skin around the tube.

Equipment for enteral (nasogastric) tube feeding

Equipment required (Fig. 4.6) consists of:

- Nasogastric tube.
- Administration set with flow regulator, with or without pump.
- A reservoir.
- Accessory equipment (stand, bag or bottle-holder).
- Liquid nutrients.

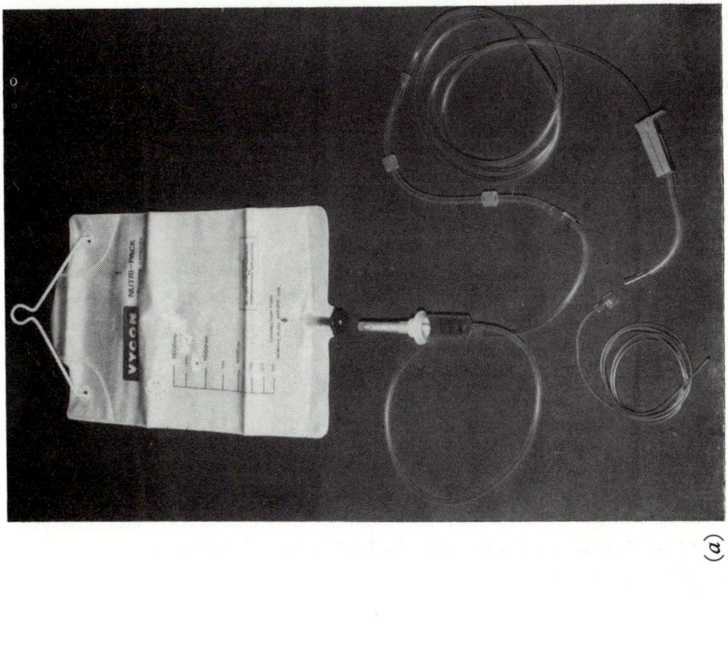

(*a*)

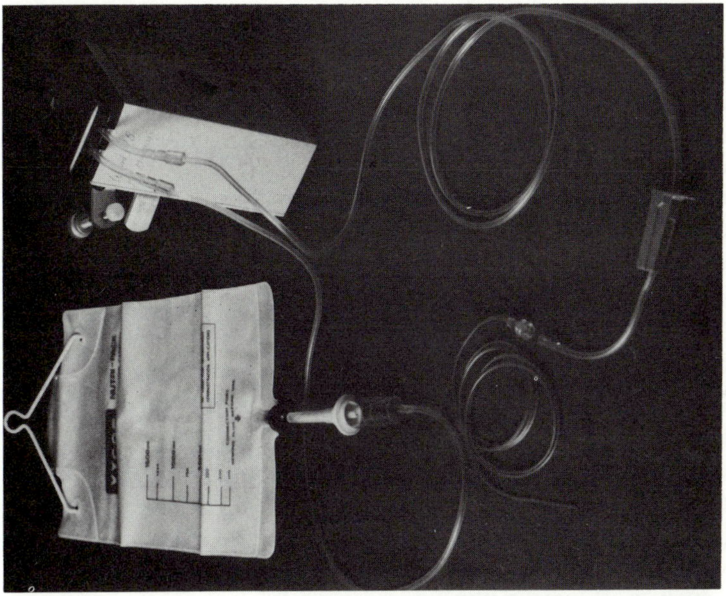

(*b*)

Fig. 4.6 (*a*) *Nasogastric enteral tube feeding system* (*Vygon*). *Nutrient reservoir, drip set with flow regulator, female luer lock end, fine bore nasogastric tube with male luer lock connector.* (*b*) *Nasogastric enteral tube feeding system incorporating flow regulator pump.*

Nasogastric tube

There are a variety of fine bore tubes available for the delivery of nutrients through the nasogastric route. These tubes are often provided by the manufacturers as a 'kit' or system (Fig. 4.6) which consists of the nasogastric tube, connectors, drip set and its flow regulator clip and the nutrient reservoir (container). Available and commonly used systems in the UK are outlined in Table 4.2. Some manufacturers of nutrient solutions for enteral feeding have now produced their own systems, which can be interchanged with minor modifications and adjustments.

In selecting equipment for enteral feeding, certain points are worthy of note.

1. Nasogastric tubes for enteral feeding must be flexible, soft and not subject to disintegration by digestive juices and radioopaque.
2. It is important for the tube to have a 'male type' luer fitting to differentiate it from the intravenous administration system and prevent incorrect use of administration sets.
3. It is important to follow the manufacturer's instructions for each system to reduce the risk of complications. Some nasogastric tubes, such as Roussel's clinifeed system, have a more rigid but flexible introducer which stops short of the tip of the tube. This is essential for this particularly fine bore and flexible tube.

Administration set and nutrient reservoir

Apart from the nasogastric tube, components of commonly used systems (Table 4.2) are similar in so far as they offer an administration set and nutrient containers. The nutrient container (or reservoir) may differ in type. Many offer a graduated plastic bag which accommodates up to 1.5 litres of liquid nutrient. These have the advantage of reducing nursing time by allowing the feeding programme to be carried out with no more than two bags. Therefore, only one or two changes are needed in 24 hours instead of several when smaller nutrient containers are used.

There are, however, two disadvantages attached to systems which offer plastic bags for their nutrient reservoir. First, the bag may have to stand for some hours with the stagnant nutrient food and there is a risk of bacterial growth if contamination has occurred. Secondly, when such a system is used, the nutrient (even when it is manufactured as a solution) has to be first transferred to the bag, with

Table 4.2 Some administration sets for enteral feeding available in UK

Designation	*Manufacturer*	*Nasogastric tube*	*Internal diameter (mm)*	*Length*	*Material*	*Systems*	*Specifications*
Duo-Tube	Argyle	Yes		102 cm	Silicone X/R	Tube alone	Weighted tip—outer PVC tube —inner silicone elastomer catheter. Bulb fitted allowing the duo tube to operate
Viomedex	Viomedex (B.D.H.)	Yes	2.3	110 cm + 140 cm	Polyurethane X/R	Yes	Hydromer coated, mercury weighted tip, female luer connection with closure cap
Nutrauxil	Viomedex (KabiVitrum)	No	—	—	—	No pump	Administration set includes drip chamber, female luer connector and bottle holder with no separate reservoir
Prima	Portex	Yes	1.1	85 cm	PVC X/R	Yes	Male luer mount, wire introducer, 1 litre bag, adaptor provided to connect to the syringe for aspiration
Clinifeed System 1	Roussel	Yes	1	70 cm	PVC X/R	Complete + pump	Male luer connection and wire introducer. 1 litre rigid plastic reservoir or $1\frac{1}{2}$ litre collapsable polythene reservoir
Clinifeed System 1/85	Roussel	Yes	1	85 cm	PVC X/R	Complete + pump	Male luer connection and wire introducer. 1 litre rigid plastic reservoir or $1\frac{1}{2}$ litre collapsable polythene reservoir
Vygon	Vygon	Yes	1	125 cm	Silicone X/R	Complete + pump	Weighted tip, male luer lock, $1\frac{1}{2}$ litre feeding bag of PVC
Vygon	Vygon	Yes	1	125 cm	PVC X/R	Complete + pump	Weighted tip, male luer lock, $1\frac{1}{2}$ litre feeding bag of PVC

increased risk of contamination. In practice, infection rarely causes difficulties. On the other hand, systems with bottle containers employ the actual bottle of nutrient as the reservoir of the system. The nutrient need not be transferred from one container to another, thus saving nursing time.

There is no particular advantage of one type of system over the other. Whichever system is selected, it must be simple, uncomplicated and one in which the nutrient container can be changed with minimum opportunities for microbial contamination and the flow rate easily adjustable to the amount required.

Accessory equipment. The drip stand and bag or bottle-holder may not appear to be an important consideration for choosing a delivery system, but the ease or difficulty with which the 'container holder' can be operated, together with durability, are factors that should be taken into account in the selection of any 'system'. This is even more important when the patient receiving enteral feeding is mobile.

Flow pumps. There appears to be some advantage in using a flow regulating pump for enteral feeding. However, the majority of hospital patients can be managed by gravity drip flow and, in these, the inclusion of a pump can complicate enteral feeding to no practical advantage.

20. Care of the Enteral Feeding System

Once the nasogastric tube, or gastrostomy or jejunostomy tube, is in position, the management of enteral feeding is almost entirely a nursing responsibility. Although enteral, compared to parenteral, feeding is relatively simple, there are still several factors which require consideration.

FEEDING

The feeding regime to be administered is determined by the patient's metabolic requirements (p. 90). The particular nutrient solutions to be given in the 24 hours are determined in conjunction with the medical and/or dietetic staff. Errors are reduced if the feeding regime is written-up and recorded in the same way as parenteral feeding, although there is no legal requirement for a medical prescription.

Clearly, it is important that the regime is adhered to, both in terms of nutrients administered and timing of administration. One of the causes of diarrhoea is too rapid administration of nutrients and, if this occurs, absorption is reduced in the gut. The feed is administered at a continuous regular rate to reduce the risk of diarrhoea. The rate is calculated according to the volume of solution to be administered in the 24-hour period. Continuous drip feeding, instead of bolus feeding, also saves nursing time and is more reliable—the feeds cannot be easily forgotten. As these feeds are being administered slowly, the temperature of the feed is unimportant as it stands at room temperature for some hours. The tube is flushed through daily with a little water to keep it patent.

Gastrostomy feeding is sometimes carried out by bolus feeding hourly or 2-hourly. It is administered slowly, and should not be cold from the refrigerator as this causes discomfort. To prevent the tube blocking, water is rinsed through the tube at the end of the feed. With a gastrostomy tube in position, air is allowed to escape from the stomach by holding the tube upright, unstoppered, before beginning feeding.

CARE OF EQUIPMENT

The nasogastric, or other, tube must be carefully fixed in position both to prevent displacement (p. 183) and to minimize discomfort of rubbing. Obviously, if there is any suspicion that the tube has become displaced, its position is checked and replaced if necessary. This is fairly unpleasant for the patient, and to be avoided, if possible, by taking care when the patient is moving, or is being moved.

The fine bore tubes, now used, are left in position for lengthy periods of time without deterioration. However, it is recommended that the administration set is changed every 24–48 hours.

21. Monitoring the Progress of Enteral Feeding

The satisfactory progress of nutrition and the prevention of complications depends on proper monitoring, involving various aspects of enteral feeding. Much of the monitoring required is the same as for parenteral feeding.

MONITORING THE INTAKE

The intake of nutrients, in terms of energy, protein and other essential components, is calculated and recorded. A chart indicating daily intake is kept to allow evaluation of the adequacy of the regime, and permit its possible adjustment. In addition, this daily recording of the intake may be used for the periodic clinical and biochemical nutritional studies. The daily water intake, together with the quantity of essential electrolytes supplied, are also recorded. Daily fluid output is measured to assess fluid balance. In the absence of abnormal losses or diarrhoea, fluid balance is easily calculated from the measured intake and the output of urine, with an allowance for insensible loss. When there are abnormal losses and/or diarrhoea, efforts should be made to calculate accurately fluid output.

PATIENT MONITORING

The patient is monitored clinically and biochemically with the object of evaluating the nutritional progress and alteration of the enteral feeding regime, when required, and preventing and treating any complications.

Clinical monitoring

The general monitoring of the patient's condition is discussed on p. 143.

There are other clinical parameters, more specifically concerned with the nutritional state and the nutritional therapy, which are monitored. These are a series of nutritional indices measured at the start of the treatment, and repeated at intervals during the progress of enteral feeding. Both the range and the frequency of these measurements depend on the initial condition of the patient, and the existing metabolic disturbances. A patient with no metabolic disease, who is given enteral feeding pre-operatively as part of the preparation for a surgical operation, requires no more than clinical and anthropometric measurements at the start of the enteral feeding therapy, and near the proposed time of surgical operation, to confirm his readiness (nutritionally) for the operation. Another patient, with a metabolic problem such as intestinal fistula, or short bowel syndrome, will require a number of parameters to be measured at frequent intervals.

As a general rule, weight is measured daily under identical conditions (p. 56). Mid-arm circumference and the skin-fold thickness are measured every 3–4 days and the results recorded. Stool frequency, volume and consistency are recorded daily. It is logical that enteral feeding relies not only on the volume of nutrient delivered, but on the fraction absorbed. The greater the volume and the frequency of faeces, the less the fraction of the given volume of nutrient available for absorption. Frequent diarrhoea in patients receiving enteral feeding means wastage of the nutrients supplied, plus loss of water and electrolytes from the patient's extracellular fluid volume. Therefore, a situation could be reached where no nutrients are absorbed and a lot of the patient's fluid is lost as well.

Biochemical parameters

Serum electrolyte and blood urea need to be estimated periodically. The frequency of their estimation depends on the metabolic seriousness of the case under review and the presence of abnormal losses and diarrhoea complicating the enteral feeding regime. Even in the absence of complications, blood urea and electrolytes are estimated every day at the start, then every 2–3 days when enteral feeding is established. Plasma proteins, albumin, transferrin and liver function tests are estimated on a regular basis in the course of enteral feeding. In patients with abnormal losses these parameters are tested every 48 hours at first, and later twice weekly. Blood glucose is also measured daily, or every 2–3 days as required. Other biochemical parameters related to trace elements, particularly calcium and magnesium, are estimated at intervals during the course of enteral feeding, particularly in patients receiving a prolonged period of treatment. In practice, a complete biochemical profile is obtained by a sample of blood which is introduced into the Auto-Analyser.

Blood count

This test is carried out regularly, the frequency depending on several factors. In the absence of complications such as occult blood loss, twice weekly testing is recommended.

Urine

The daily volume of urine passed is recorded. Urinary electrolyte and urea estimations (of 24 hour specimens) is carried out, the frequency depending on the general metabolic state of the patient. In many cases these need to be done every 3–4 days. When there is a possibility of glucose intolerance, then urinary biochemistry is carried out daily. It is good practice in the ward to carry out daily glucose and ketone testing of the urine and to evaluate urinary specific gravity, or osmolality.

TECHNICAL MONITORING

One of the purposes of monitoring is to ensure the adequacy of the intake of nutrients, which is dependent on the efficiency of the method used for the delivery of the food into the alimentary tract and the prevention of complications.

Once the nasogastric feeding tube is passed, and its correct position checked radiologically, it is simple to check the position of the tube at regular intervals. In some conditions, such as obstructuve lesions of the oesophagus or upper stomach, the tube can be displaced during vomiting and regurgitation. Delivery of nutrients into the oesophagus is then attended by more vomiting, particularly if there is an obstruction.

If a flow regulator pump is used, the running of the pump is checked at least every time the nutrient container is changed.

In gastrostomy and jejunostomy tube feeding, the skin around the tube is checked regularly for skin irritation and excoriation, which can lead to discomfort and infection.

22. Complications of Enteral Feeding: Prevention and Treatment

An important aspect in the management of patients receiving enteral feeding is the prevention and treatment of complications. The fact that enteral feeding is less complicated in its technique, and simpler in its monitoring, than intravenous feeding, should not create a false impression that it has no risk of danger, or is without its complications. Familiarity with potential complications of enteral feeding is important so as to prevent them developing. Complications must always be recognized, recorded and reported.

Complications of enteral feeding may be grouped under (1) complications related to the technique of feeding; and (2) metabolic complications and those related to the nutrient intake.

COMPLICATIONS OF THE TECHNIQUE OF FEEDING

The incidence of these complications is dependent on the administration system and the route of delivery.

Misplacement and displacement of the nasogastric tube

Occasionally, difficulty is encountered in introducing the nasogastric tube through the nose and pharynx. In some patients suffering from obstructive lesions of the oesophagus, there is considerable difficulty in achieving the passage of the tube. Even when the endoscopic method of placement is used, there may still be difficulty in passing the tube. These patients are nourished intravenously until the obstruction is relieved. However, displacement of the nasogastric tube can occur during vomiting or coughing. If there is any suspicion that this has occurred, the correct position is checked again.

Blockage of the tube

A fine bore tube can become blocked. This is prevented by using the correct system for a particular nutrient solution, and by continuous flow of the solution. From time-to-time the tube is flushed through with clear fluid.

Gastrostomy and jejunostomy tube leakage

This complication occurs particularly when there is a reduction in peristalsis, leading to stagnation of nutrients in the gastrointestinal tract. When the nutrient solution is introduced continuously, but slowly, this is less likely to occur as even when there is a reduction in rate of peristalsis the alimentary tract is not overloaded.

Nasopharyngeal ulcer, sore throat, in nasogastric tube feeding

Many patients may feel discomfort at the beginning. Some complain of a sore throat and a few may develop nasopharyngeal inflammation and ulceration.

Gentle introduction of the nasogastric tube, and prevention of dehydration, reduces the likelihood of a sore throat or inflammation developing, and progressing to ulcers. A throat swab is taken for microbiological studies when inflammation, infection and ulceration is present. An antiseptic and mild analgesic is then given as a mouth wash and for gargling. The use of a fine bore tube made of non-irritant material reduces the risk of this complication.

Gastric erosion and ulcers

This complication sometimes occurs with nasogastric, or gastrostomy, tubes. Malaena stool or aspiration of coffee-ground fluid from the stomach point to this complication, which is noted and reported to the medical staff.

Oesophagitis and stricture

Passage of a nasogastric tube into the stomach can result in incompetence of the cardia, gastro-oesophageal reflux, oesophagitis and stricture. This complication was common in the early days when a rubber tube was employed for nasogastric tube aspiration and feeding. At present, the incidence of oesophagitis and stricture is low, but if heartburn and reflux occurs this is noted and reported and appropriate antireflux medication given.

Aspiration and inhalation of nutrients

Apart from misplacement and displacement of the feeding tube, with accidental introduction of nutrient into the trachea (an accident which should never occur), regurgitation may occur followed by aspiration of nutrient solutions into the bronchial tree.

This complication particularly occurs in the elderly, emaciated patient to whom the nutrients are introduced as a bolus or too rapidly, and in unconscious patients. The upwards displacement of the nasogastric tube from the stomach into the oesophagus, and introduction of nutrient into the oesophagus, may also occasion this complication. Patients with severe mid- or high-oesophageal obstruction, even with the tube in the correct position, may have aspiration of saliva or regurgitate nutrients. Such patients are monitored with particular regard to their respiratory system and the development of 'wet chest'.

METABOLIC COMPLICATIONS AND NUTRIENT INTAKE

These complications are due to the side-effects of the nutrients or the metabolic disturbances of tube feeding.

Nausea and vomiting

This complication may be caused by:

- a too rapid and large volume of solution administered, but continuous regular flow and use of a pump usually prevents it happening;

- high osmolality and concentration of the nutrient solution. Dilution of the nutrients and a gradual increase to the full required amount and concentration over a few days, prevent nausea and vomiting caused by hyperosmolar nutrients.

Maxolon syrup, 10 ml three times daily, may be helpful in many cases.

Diarrhoea

A concentrated hyperosmolar nutrient solution introduced into the gastrointestinal tract acts similarly to osmotic purgatives in producing diarrhoea. Diarrhoea is probably the commonest type of complication and, in the majority of cases, is due to a hyperosmolar nutrient solution given as a bolus or administered too rapidly.

In some instances, diarrhoea is induced or promoted by drugs (such as antibiotics) which patients are taking for an independent illness while receiving enteral nutrition. A few people are lactose intolerant and have diarrhoea if the feed contains lactose.

When diarrhoea occurs in patients having enteral feeding, the amount and type of nutrient, its composition, osmolality and the way it is administered is considered. It is suggested that solutions of high osmolality increase the incidence of diarrhoea. The use of large carbohydrate molecules (such as in Caloreen) and whole protein, rather than amino acids, is recommended (Allison *et al.*, 1979). When diarrhoea persists (in spite of the above mentioned precautions) and providing it is not infective, Codeine phosphate 30–60 mg twice or three times a day is of great help.

Hyperosmolar state and osmotic diuresis

These complications are essentially due to the administration of a hyperosmolar solution into the gastrointestinal tract, which in turn is absorbed into the blood. This causes an increase in plasma osmolality and hyperosmolar renal filtrate, which prevents the reabsorption of water in the renal tubules and results in a diuresis and disturbance of water balance. These cause dehydration, hyperglycaemia and uraemia.

In some instances, patients have an abnormal glucose tolerance (e.g. following injury) and develop hyperglycaemia and glycosuria, particularly when a high concentration of glucose is administered. Urine tests, similar to those for diabetics, and daily blood sugar testing are carried out and insulin given in hyperglycaemia, the dose being adjusted on a sliding scale according to the blood and urine test results. Dehydration is prevented by carefully monitoring the fluid balance and the plasma and urine osmolality and taking appropriate action.

Uraemia

In many cases, uraemia is an expression of dehydration or imbalance of calorie or nitrogen intake (i.e. too little calorie for too much protein). Blood and urine urea (24 hour) is checked frequently in such cases and the dietary imbalance corrected accordingly.

Deficiency complications

Enteral feeding, particularly when used as a longterm feeding method and when complicated by diarrhoea, hyperosmolar state or inadequate attention to intake, may be attended by deficiencies. Deficiency hypoprothrombinaemia, anaemia, folic acid and essential fatty acid deficiency cases have been reported. Generally, these complications are rare in ordinary hospital patients when nutritional support is not of a long duration. Nevertheless their existence must be kept in mind.

REFERENCES

Allison S.P., Walford S., Todorovic V., Elliot E.T. (1979). Practical aspects of nutritional support. In *Developments in Clinical Nutrition.* (Johnston I.D.A., Lee H.A., eds.). Symposium held October, 1978. Tunbridge Wells: MCS Consultants.

Hayward J. (1975). *Information : a Prescription Against Pain.* London: Royal College of Nursing.

Johnson J.E. (1976). Stress reduction through sensation information. In *Stress and Anxiety 2* (Sarason I.G., Spielberger, C.D., eds.), New York: Halstad Press.

Jones D.C. (1975). *Food for Thought.* London: Royal College of Nursing.

FURTHER READING

Allison S.P. (1981). Fine bore tube feeding. Second European Congress of Parenteral and Enteral Nutrition, September, 1980. *Acta Chirurgica Scandinavica. Suppl.*; **507**.

Janes E. (1982). Oral nutritional supplements. *Nursing* (Oxford); **2**(5): 126–127, 137.

Johnston, I.D.A., Lee H.A. (1979). *Developments in Clinical Nutrition.* Symposium held at Royal College of Physicians, London, October, 1978. Tunbridge Wells: MCS Consultants.

Jones B.J.M., Payne S., Silk D.B.A. (1980). Indications for pump-assisted enteral feeding. *Lancet*; **1**: 1057–1058.

Kagawa-Busby K.S., Heltkemper M.M., Hansen B.C., Hanson R.L., Vanderburg V.V. (1980). Effects of diet temperature on tolerance of enteral feedings. *Nurs. Res.*; **29**: 276–280.

Michigan Nurses Association—Curn Project (1981). *Using Research to Improve Nursing Practice: Reducing Diarrhoea in Tube-fed Patients.* New York: Grune and Stratton.

Rombeau J.L., Barot L.R. (1981). Enteral nutritional therapy. *Surg. Clin. of N. America*; **61**(3): 605–620.

Tredgar J., Bazin C., Dickerson J.W.T. (1981). Nasogastric tube feeding. A survey to investigate current practices and attitudes of dietitians. *J. of Hum. Nutr.*; **35**: 118–122.

Woolfson A.M.J., Ricketts C.R., Hardy S.M., Sadur M.D., Pollard B.J., Allison S.P. (1976). Prolonged nasogastric tube feeding in critically ill and surgical patients. *Post-Graduate Medical Journal*; **52**: 678–682.

SECTION V

Topics

This section discusses a few topics in artificial feeding. These are specialized subjects, and all that is attempted here is to give an introduction to them. This being so, a general view of each is provided. For those more concerned with aspects of nutrition selected references are provided at the end of this section.

23. Nutrition and Cancer

Cancer may be considered as a group of diseases with the common characteristic of invasion and destruction of normal tissues and their replacement by abnormal cells. Although there are many types of malignant tumours (commonly referred to as cancer), they all share the common property of depending on the bodies 'pool' of nutrients, without contributing to it or subserving any function in return.

Nutrition is concerned with cancer in several ways, of which the following are important:

1. Cancer can develop as a result of carcinogens being introduced into the body in food, or as an additive. (This aspect is not considered here.)

2. Cancer can affect the nutritional status, and often leads to malnutrition.

3. Nutritional deficiencies can result from the effect of treatment and, therefore, malnutrition can be the direct result of the deleterious effects of specific cancer therapy.

EFFECT OF CANCER ON NUTRITIONAL STATE

Cancer may influence the nutritional state in a number of ways. Some tumours, particularly those of the alimentary tract, directly affect the ingestion, digestion or absorption of food. It is not difficult to realize that an obstructive cancer of the oesophagus can, after a time, cause malnutrition due to lack of ingestion. In other instances, a tumour may lead to obstruction or cause fistulae, which in turn prevent absorption of nutrients or increases nutrient loss from the body.

Cancer tissues may, by their metabolism, affect the nutritional state and result in malnutrition. Tumour tissues utilize amino acids from the body 'pool' (p. 14) for incorporation into their own proteins. For as long as food intake is adequately maintained, and the metabolic necessities are available, cancer tissues are provided with nutrients from that source. If nutrients for cancer tissue metabolism are not available in food intake, then they have to be derived from the tissues and reserves of the host, who, therefore, develops malnutrition.

Some cancer patients suffer from anorexia, loss of taste and smell, with consequent reduction in food intake.

In some cases of cancer the metabolic processes are directly interfered with by extensive involvement of the part of the brain principally concerned with metabolism.

The sum total of the cancer and nutritional state is malnutrition, which in extreme cases is clinically recognized by cachexia.

INFLUENCE OF CANCER TREATMENT AND NUTRITION

All therapeutic modalities for cancer have a direct or indirect influence on nutrition.

Surgery

A surgical operation is attended by an increase in metabolism (p. 38) proportional to the extent and the severity of the operation.

Radiotherapy

Various forms of radiation used in the treatment of cancer are all associated with nutritional problems—some of which are apparent in an early stage of treatment. In some patients, nausea, vomiting and loss of appetite are severe enough to affect food intake and lead to loss of weight and malnutrition. Those treated for upper alimentary tract cancers have additional causes for malnutrition, or at least under-nourishment, due to a sore throat, lack of appetite and oesophagitis. Those receiving radiotherapy to the upper abdomen may suffer from diarrhoea and malabsorption, in addition to the effect of reduced intake.

Chemotherapy

All cytotoxic agents used in cancer chemotherapy have side-effects which adversely affect food intake or absorption of nutrients. The degree to which the nutritional state is compromised in cancer chemotherapy is dependent on the drugs administered and the susceptibility of an individual.

Cancer patients are especially prone to develop malnutrition due to their illness, as elaborated above. They are, in addition, subject to further deterioration of their nutritional state due to their specific cancer treatment.

NUTRITIONAL MANAGEMENT OF CANCER PATIENTS

Having discussed the effects of cancer and its treatment on the nutritional state, it is important to consider the ways in which cancer sufferers may be helped.

Cancer is a common condition affecting a vast number of people in any community. A number of cancer patients in the terminal phase of their illness are nutritionally severely deficient. Some become cachectic, a few however are hospitalized primarily for their cancer treatment. In all these patients, nutritional assessment is carried out. It may reasonably be wondered how far this assessment should be pursued. The experience of those who deal with great numbers of cancer patients in hospital (and are seriously interested in the nutritional aspect of their patient's care) indicate that there is no necessity (except for scientific data collection) to submit patients to many elaborate tests (p. 52) to assess their nutritional status. They can be assessed, for practical purposes, by simple tests consisting of clinical examination, weight and anthropometric measurements and routine blood biochemistry and blood count. There is little doubt that with these minimal tests and nursing observations and records of food intake, cancer patients can be judged either under- or malnourished.

When radiotherapy and/or chemotherapy is the therapeutic choice, it is even more important that food intake is recorded and nutritional support given. Once the necessity of providing artificial nutritional support is determined, then the method of feeding may be decided upon (p. 163).

24. Home Parenteral Nutrition

The experience and the widespread acceptance of parenteral nutrition as a therapeutic method for hospital patients is responsible for the development of home parenteral feeding (HPN), which has now become a practical reality and a significant advance in the life-support system. In effect, the theoretical background of HPN is the natural progression and extension of the hospital parenteral nutrition to a specific group of patients in whom the continuous persistence of their intestinal failure make them subjects for prolonged intravenous feeding. This is best undertaken in the normal environment of a patient's home. This not only obviates the necessity for prolonged hospitalization, with all the institutionalization effects, but is also a less expensive undertaking.

Home parenteral nutrition is a specialized subject and its methods and applications are beyond the scope of this book. However, a general view is given that should be useful for all interested in artificial feeding.

In North America HPN has been used since the 1970s, and hundreds have been helped and artificially fed in their own homes. In the UK, HPN has been slower to start, but a few centres have now reported their experience; each centre having only one or two patients—totalling some 10–12 patients in all.

The indications for HPN essentially focus around the intestinal failure and the conditions causing it. Crohn's disease heads the list of indications both in a North American and UK series. Multiple fistulae and short-bowel syndrome, arising as a result of Crohn's disease, are also included. Total bowel resection constitutes about one-third of cases in the Canadian series, which may be considered as the first centre to use HPN in patients with total bowel resection, therefore needing permanent parenteral feeding. An American, and at least one European, series show a number of patients with cancer having chemotherapy or radiotherapy and receiving longterm parenteral nutrition at home, or outside hospital.

In many patients, HPN has been the continuation of a hospital's total parenteral feeding and, when patients are first considered for HPN, it is hoped that they will be cases for prolonged or longterm parenteral nutrition therapy, but not permanent ones. Indeed, the ideal indications for HPN are those who can be gradually weaned off artificial feeding and resume oral food intake.

Since metabolism and the patient's life depends on prolonged or permanent total parenteral nutrition the continuing delivery of the nutrients into the blood stream is obviously essential. There has, therefore, been considerable research into the techniques and methods of catheter placement, its care and the material used in its manufacture which best serve the purposes of HPN. A subclavian vein is most commonly used for the catheter insertion by employing the cut-down technique and subcutaneous tunnelling (p. 112). Bilateral subclavian venography is usually performed to determine the optimal site for the catheter insertion, which is then carried out in an operating theatre, preferably under radiological surveillance. The catheter itself is normally made of silicon rubber. The delivery system for HPN is generally similar to that used in hospital and consists of catheter, infusion system with a mini pump and nutrient container. Nutritional intake can be given at intervals, with much of it administered overnight to allow the patient to live as normal a life as possible. The intravenous catheter is filled with heparinized saline and closed with a two-way tap between feeds.

One aspect of HPN that has attracted attention and influenced the selection of patients, particularly in North America, is the mental attitude of the patients and their aptitude to undertake the task of administration. Patients using HPN have to be taught to undertake the care of the catheter, the site of exit and the infusion system. The formulation of the regime is made while patients are in hospital, on the basis of remaining in positive nitrogen balance, and the given diet is then prescribed for home feeding. Nutrients have to be delivered to the patient's home, and regular biochemistry checks and nutritional efficiency tests performed. It is, therefore, clear that HPN is a viable method in the life-support system for a selected group of patients who not only survive, but also have a useful and reasonable quality of life. For a few selected patients, HPN is a worthwhile undertaking by centres with a back-up team and coordinated facilities. Even for the cost conscious, HPN is invaluable, particularly in those who can eventually be weaned-off total parenteral nutrition. The cost of keeping a patient in hospital on longterm total parenteral nutrition is much more expensive to implement than HPN.

25. Artificial Feeding in Children

The field of artificial nutrition in neonates and children is discussed in detail in other publications, so it is only intended here to merely introduce some ideas which may help in recognizing some of the important elements.

A great deal of what is written in this book is also applicable to babies and children. However, adaptations must be made to take into account the differing nutritional requirements of children and the technical difficulties associated with their small size.

Nutritional requirements are greater in relation to size, and somewhat different in children as compared to adults. The metabolic rate in children is higher and, therefore, the energy requirements per kg body weight is greater. In planning their intake allowance has to be made to allow normal growth, in addition to requirements for replacement and repair of tissue. This is particularly important in pre-term and young babies at a critical stage in growth and development, when deficiencies are not compensated by adequate feeding at a later stage. Thus, protein needs are increased and certain amino acids, which are formed in adequate amounts by adults, are essential in the diet of children. (This is discussed further by MacMahon, James *et al.*, 1980.)

Technically, the small size of the veins increases the difficulty of setting up a satisfactory parenteral feeding system, and the smaller the child or infant the more difficult the procedure. Similar methods for placement of the venous catheter are used as in adults. However, Shaw (1980) recommends the insertion of a fine catheter into a peripheral vein (preferably a scalp vein), which is then advanced carefully through the venous sytem until the tip is positioned in the right atrium. The position is checked radiologically and the procedure carried out without removing the baby from the incubator. Infants, particularly premature or sick babies, lose heat rapidly and may become hypothermic if exposed to normal ward temperatures for any length of time during cannulation. Precautions to prevent this are always taken.

COMPLICATIONS

Children receiving enteral or parenteral feeding are subject to the same complications that occur in adults and similar action is therefore taken to minimize risk and prevent complications. Neonates are particularly at risk of succumbing to any infection which may occur through the enteral or parenteral route.

In addition, difficulties can arise because of the very nature of an infant or toddler. In the infant, it is critically important to regulate the fluid intake and accurately adjust the fluid balance. Children are much more sensitive to fluid and electrolyte disturbances than adults. While the 5 ml of water used to flush through a nasogastric tube is of little importance in an adult, it is a sizeable amount for a small baby. To ensure accurate fluid intake, a micro-drip set with a burette is used in intravenous feeding, allowing very accurate control of the rate of intake.

As a baby grows into a toddler, mobility increases and problems now arise in maintaining an artificial feeding system against prying hands. To prevent the nasogastric tube being pulled out, or disruption of the dressing over the intravenous cannula insertion site, some restraint will be needed. The child must be restrained in such a way that he/she is prevented from disrupting the feeding system, but nevertheless is moderately comfortable. This is simple in the very ill child, but is more difficult as the condition improves. The involvement of the parent is very important at this stage as they can hold and play with their child so that he is happy and relaxed, and help stop any interference with the nutritional system.

Communication to gain the necessary cooperation to carry out any of the procedures involved in enteral or parenteral feeding will vary with the age and understanding of the child. A tiny baby can readily be restrained to allow procedures to be performed. It is the parents who need the explanation of what is going on, and need considerable support and help from the nursing staff to help them accept what is happening to their child.

With a toddler, however, the carrying out of any procedure is much more difficult as he will not yet understand the explanation given, but realizes that something is going on. The child may have considerable strength to resist, and parental involvement becomes very important, perhaps, but not necessarily, in helping to restrain him, but certainly in helping to comfort him afterwards.

As the child develops in understanding, a clear explanation should be given as to what is happening to him, what it will feel like, and what he must do. The language used and the detail given is adjusted according to the understanding of the child. It has been found that children are helped by play to deal with the events taking place in hospital. A doll going through the same procedure, with the same equipment, helps prepare the child for the event to come, or to come to terms with any unpleasant past events. Even very young children are helped in this way.

Any child in hospital, but particularly the infant or child on artificial feeding, is at risk of deprivation of contact and play. Close physical contact is needed by all children, and this should preferably be provided by the parents. They must be encouraged, as far as possible, to hold and cuddle their child, be involved in his care and spend as much time as possible with him, thus maintaining the parent–child bond. Mobility is somewhat limited when a child is receiving artificial feeding, and this can restrict the ability to receive a varying sensory input and to play. Both are important for normal intellectual development to occur and it is important to ensure that they are supplied.

If the hospital is to 'do the patient no harm' (Florence Nightingale) these are essential requirements. Once the child's condition improves, and he becomes more mobile, toys, games and even school can be brought to him, or he can be taken to them, along with the artificial feeding system. The company of other children is also of value in developing social skills.

26. Organization of Nutritional Support

Throughout this book it has been pointed out that artificial nutrition requires organization with regard to the planning, technical application and assessment of its efficiency. In effect, the success and the smooth running of nutritional therapy depends on the cooperation of many individuals of differing disciplines, who may be referred to as the nutritional team.

A team of people trained in different aspects of artificial nutrition can, by their wealth of available expertise, offer considerable benefits to patients requiring nutritional support. Undertaking any form of therapy by a team has much to recommend, but it also has its shortcomings. Nevertheless, when organizing nutritional support within an institution, a department, or even a ward, the concept of the nutritional team must be considered. The size and function of a team and its individual members will require more thought and discussion.

SIZE OF THE TEAM

The size and constituent members of a nutritional support team can vary greatly, depending on the local requirements, available facilities and the scope of duties assigned to them. A physician or surgeon, nurse and dietician are regarded as essential. They decide upon the necessity of nutritional support for a patient, plan the regime, dispense the nutrients and monitor the progress of the treatment and its effect on the patient. A small organization can operate effectively within a ward, but access to the expertise of other specialists, such as pharmacists, and knowledge of nutritional products and available additives are essential. The assistance of other medical and nursing staff concerned with the day-to-day management of the patient is also of benefit. In effect, this type of organization can realistically undertake the nutritional care in many small departments whose main activity is not concerned with nutrition. Medical or surgical wards of a hospital accommodate many types of patient who may well fall within this category, and can be nutritionally organized by such a small team.

In other circumstances, the team can include a much larger representation from various specialities. It is, for instance, possible to form a team whose constituent members are a physician, surgeon, dietician, nurse nutritionist, pharmacist, biochemist, etc. This type of team may then undertake the responsibility for artificial feeding in a large district general hospital, and there is no doubt that such groups can provide excellent nutritional advice to their area or hospital. However, the difficulties that can arise are:

1. The adaptation of nutritional therapy within the overall treatment of patients. That is, the nutritional team may not fully appreciate the entire clinical picture of a patient and may look at the nutritional problems in isolation.

2. The clinician in charge of patients may not fully appreciate the function of a nutritional team and may not cooperate with them. Therefore, if the clinician is not involved in the inauguration of a team, he may not wish them to be involved with his patients.

3. Patient management may fall into the hands of different teams, each with expertise of its own. There may therefore be a danger of fragmentation of the management of patient care.

FUNCTIONS OF THE TEAM

A small team consisting of the doctor, who is usually in charge of the patient, a ward sister and dietician can function most satisfactorily in a medical or surgical ward. This ward care team can not only see the nutritional problem, but also plan and apply the nutritional therapy. They also have the definite advantage of knowing the whole of a patient's problems, so as to design a nutritional programme within the overall therapeutic management of that patient. If this be the organization and the function of a team, the help and assistance of other specialists may be obtained.

A larger team may function in two different ways:

1. They can act as advisers on the nutritional problems of patients and all aspects of the artificial feeding, including details of the type of artificial feeding and its technical aspects. They are in a position to act as advisers and planners to large areas, the whole of a hospital or district, but they do not participate in the practical application, although they may teach others.
2. A large team may act both as an adviser and assist with day-to-day practical management of the nutritional problems, in cooperation with the ward staff.

The key to the organization of nutritional support is flexibility and consideration of local requirements, and the type of nutritional support available. Parenteral and enteral feeding are not exclusive alternatives, but two modalities which can be used for the nutritional support of a patient at different times, either separately or together. Whatever organization is envisaged to undertake nutritional therapy at ward level, nurse participation is obviously very great and the ward sister is ultimately responsible for patient management. For those receiving nutritional support, this must include the nursing aspects of nutritional therapy.

New members of staff must be aware of the routine and procedures concerned with the nutritional management of patients. Therefore, a teaching programme on all aspects of artificial nutrition should be organized, using the expertise of the nutritional team in its planning.

REFERENCES—FURTHER READING

Nutrition and Cancer

Brennan M.F. (1981). Total parenteral nutrition in the management of the cancer patient. Second European Congress on Parenteral and Enteral

Nutrition Symposia held September, 1980. *Acta. Chirurgica Scandinavica. Suppl.*; **507**: 428–434.
Butler, J.H. (1980). Nutrition and cancer: a review of the literature. *Cancer Nursing*; **3**: 131–136.
Copeland E.M., Dudrick S.J. (1976). Nutritional aspects of cancer. *Curr. Probl. Cancer*; **1**(3): 1–51.
Dickerson J.W.T. (1981). The role of enteral nutrition in malignant disease. Second European Congress on Parenteral and Enteral Nutrition Symposia held September, 1980. *Acta. Chirurgica Scandinavica. Suppl.*; **507**: 422–427
Dickerson J.W.T. (1981). Nutrition and the patient with cancer. *Proc. Nutr. Soc.*; **40**(1): 31–35.
Dickerson J.W.T., Tredger J.A. (1978). Nutrition and the cancer patient. In *Oncology for Nurses and Health Care Professionals. Vol. 2, Care and Support* (Tiffany R., ed.). London: George Allen and Unwin.
Dionigi R., Campani M. (1981). Nutritional and immunological abnormalities in malignant disease. Second European Congress on Parenteral and Enteral Nutrition Symposia held September, 1980. *Acta. Chirurgica Scandinavica. Suppl.*; **507**: 435–474.
Ivey S.P. (1982). Nutrition and cancer patients. *Nursing* (Oxford); **2**(5): 129–132.
Janes E. (1981). The nutritional problems of patients with cancer and nursing approaches to resolve them. In *Cancer Nursing Update: 2nd International Cancer Nursing Conference* (Tiffany R., ed.). London: Bailliere Tindall.
Shils M.E. (1979). Diet and nutrition as modifying factors in tumour development. *Med. Clin. of N. America*; **63**(5): 1027–1041.
Shils M.E. (1979). Nutritional problems induced by cancer. *Med. Clin. of N. America*; **63**(5): 1009–1025.

Home Parenteral Nutrition

Hardy G., Kiepert D.R. (1981). The role of the pharmaceutical industry in home parenteral nutrition. Second European Congress on Parenteral and Enteral Nutrition Symposia held September, 1980. *Acta. Chirurgica Scandinavica, Suppl.*; **507**: 121–127.
Irving M. (1981). Home parenteral nutrition in the United Kingdom. Second European Congress on Parenteral and Enteral Nutrition Symposia held September, 1980. *Acta. Chirurgica Scandinavica, Suppl.*; **507**: 140–142.
Jarnum S., Ladefoged K. (1981). European experience of home parenteral nutrition. Second European Congress on Parenteral and Enteral Nutrition Symposia held September, 1980. *Acta. Chirurgica Scandinavica. Suppl.*; **507**: 128–139.
Lees C.D., Steiger E., Hooley R.A., Montague N., Srp, F., LaMantia S., Gulledge A.D., Gipson W.T., Frame C. (1981). Home parenteral nutrition. Second European Congress of Parenteral and Enteral Nutrition Symposia held September, 1980. *Acta. Chirurgica Scandinavica. Suppl.*; **507**: 113–120.
Lees C.D., Steiger E., Hooley R.A., Montague N. *et al.* (1981). Home

parenteral nutrition. *Surgical Clinics of North America*; **61**(3): 621–633.
Solassol C., Joyeux H. (1976). Ambulatory parenteral nutrition. In *Total Parenteral Nutrition* (Fischer J.E., ed.). Boston: Little Brown.

Artificial feeding in children

MacMahon R.A., James B., Shaw P., Hendry P., Yu V., Bornstein J. (1980). Intravenous solutions in parenteral nutrition. Second European Congress on Parenteral and Enteral Nutrition Symposia held September, 1980. *Acta. Chirurgica Scandinavica. Suppl.*; **507**: 248–257.
Shaw J.C.L. (1980). Technical problems in parenteral nutrition of the premature infant. Second European Congress on Parenteral and Enteral Nutrition Symposia held September, 1980. *Acta. Chirurgica Scandinavica. Suppl.*; **507**: 258–268.
Coran, A.G. (1980). Nutritional support of the paediatric surgical patient. In *Paediatric Surgery* (Holder T.M., Aschcraft K.W., eds.). Philadelphia: W.B. Saunders.
Frayer W., Redo S.F. (1981). Nutrition in the paediatric patient. In *Surgical Nutrition* (Yarborough M.F., Curreri P.W., eds.). Edinburgh: Churchill Livingstone.
Johnston I.D.A., ed. (1978). Advances in parenteral nutrition. Section VI. In *Parenteral Nutrition in Paediatrics*. Lancaster: M.T.P. Press.
Wilmore D.W., Dudrick S.J. (1968). Growth and development of an infant receiving all nutrients exclusively by vein. *JAMA*; **203**: 860–864.

Organization of Nutritional Support

Blackburn G.L., Bothe A., Lahey M.A. (1981). Organization and administration of a nutrition support service. *Surg. Clin. of N. America*; **61**(3): 709–719.
Englert DeA. (1981). The role of the nurse in intravenous hyperalimentation in the United States. Second European Congress on Parenteral and Enteral Nutrition Symposia held September, 1980. *Acta. Chirurgica Scandinavica. Suppl.*; **507**: 298–313.
Janes E.M.H. (1981). The importance of follow-up in the nutritional care of the cancer patient. Second European Congress on Parenteral and Enteral Nutrition Symposia held September, 1980. *Acta. Chirurgica Scandinavica. Suppl.*; **507**: 162–166.
Johnston I.D.A. (1981). The relevance of nutritional care to the hospital patient. Second European Congress on Parenteral and Enteral Nutrition Symposia held September, 1980. *Acta. Chirurgica Scandinavica. Suppl.*; **507**: 289–291.
Keersmaecker L.De. (1981). Pharmacy role in a total parenteral nutrition therapy—methods and equipment. Second European Congress on Parenteral and Enteral Nutrition Symposia held September, 1980. *Acta. Chirurgica Scandinavica. Suppl.*; **507**: 375–382.
Stordy B.J. (1981). The psychological importance of nutrients and food. Second European Congress on Parenteral and Enteral Nutrition Symposia

held September, 1980, *Acta Chirurgica Scandinavica. Suppl.*; **507**: 151–154.

Tredgar J. (1982). Feeding the patient—a team effort. *Nursing* (Oxford); **2**(4): 92–93.

Tweedle D.E.F. (1981). Organising nutritional support. Second European Congress on Parenteral and Enteral Nutrition Symposia held September, 1980. *Acta. Chirurgica Scandinavica. Suppl.*; **507**: 292–297.

Index